Props for Yoga

A Guide to Iyengar Yoga Practice with Props

Volume III: Inverted *āsana-s* - *Viparīta Sthiti*

by

Eyal Shifroni

Props for Yoga

A Guide to Iyengar Yoga Practice with Props

Volume III: Inverted *āsana-s - Viparīta Sthiti*

Eyal Shifroni, Ph.D.

Based on the teachings of
Yogacharya B.K.S. Iyengar, Geeta S. Iyengar and Prashant S. Iyengar
at the Ramamani Iyengar Memorial Yoga Institute (RIMYI), Pune, India.

Text Editing Sivan Goldhirsh

Models Ravit Moar, Eleanor Jacobovitz, Anat Rachmel, Michael Sela, Inbar Shifroni & Eyal Shifroni

Photography Yul Shifroni (www.yulshift.com)

Photo Editing and Figures Shira Katz

Graphic Design Asaf Goral

Props Illustrations Kym Ben-Yaakov

ISBN 978-965-92519-3-3

Acknowledgments and Gratitude

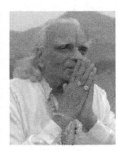

1918 - 2014

The source of all the knowledge presented in this guide is my Guru, *Yogācharya* B.K.S Iyengar, the founder of the Iyengar Yoga method. Since he was my Guru in yoga I refer to him as Guruji Iyengar. The use of props in yoga practice was introduced by Guruji Iyengar. The various apparatus which he invented and adapted over the years were created to enrich practice and to enable every person to benefit from the gift of Yoga. It is already more than two years since Guruji Iyengar has left us, nevertheless, every day, when I return to my Yoga mat, I remember him with great appreciation, gratitude and love, and I thank him from the bottom of my heart for the precious gift of Yoga he had given to us. I feel that when I practice he still lives inside of me, and his sharp authoritative voice echoing in my head, calling me to improve my practice, to be more attentive, to dive deeper to the heart of every *āsana* without any compromise. I feel that as long we continue to practice seriously, as he taught us, he will continue to live in our hearts. I wish to express my deep admiration and gratitude to Guruji Iyengar, not only as a personal teacher, but also for making yoga accessible to millions worldwide.

I wish to thank Prashant and Geeta Iyengar for their guidance and inspiration in their teaching in RIMYI[1].

I have been very fortunate to have come across many inspiring teachers who have shared their deep knowledge with me and who have shed light on Yoga in general and on the use of props in particular. They are too many to list their names here. However, I am indebted to each and every one of them and wish to express my deep gratitude to them all. I have done my best to convey to you readers the rich knowledge transmitted to me by all these talented and knowledgeable teachers. If, however, any inaccuracy or mistake is found in my presentation it is my sole responsibility.

Many thanks to my friends and colleagues, Michael Sela and Sivan Goldhirsh, who went through the text over and over again and contributed substantially to its correctness, clarity and flow. I wish to express deep appreciation for their collaboration on this project.

Special thanks to Jawahar Bangera, a very senior teacher from Mumbai, for reading the manuscript of this book, for correcting and improving the text

[1] Ramāmaṇi Iyengar Memorial Yoga Institute – the home and teaching site of the Iyengars in Pune, India.

v

and mostly for encouraging me to continue with this hard (but rewarding) work. I wish to thank also Karin Freschi, an Iyengar yoga teacher from Italy, a dear friend and colleague, for reading the text and for giving many insightful comments and corrections.

Thanks to all the teachers at the Iyengar Yoga Zichron-Ya'akov center who contributed many beneficial ideas and feedback; special thanks go to Ravit Moar, Anat Rachmel and Michael Sela for spending so many hours modeling for the photos in this guide. As yoga teachers, your contribution goes much beyond mere modeling – you gave many insights and ideas that improved the contents of this guide. Ohad Nachtomy and Eden Gershon also helped with the photography.

I extend many thanks to my students, who helped testing and developing new ideas of using props during classes and workshops. Their willingness to try out these ideas and their enthusiastic feedback encouraged me to write this guide.

And, last but not least, thanks to my family members – my sweet daughters, Yul Shifroni who took most of the photographs for this book and Inbar Shifroni (a yoga teacher in her own right) who modeled for some of the photos. I am always indebted to my beloved wife, Hagit, for her continuous love and support which made this guide (and many other things) possible.

Preface to the 3ʳᵈ volume

This is the 3ʳᵈ volume in the *Props for Yoga* series, which provides a comprehensive description on the usage of props in the Iyengar method. Volume I focused on standing *āsana-s* and Volume II focused on sitting *āsana-s* and forward bends. This volume focuses on inverted *āsana-s*.

I always liked being upside-down; at the age of 10, in my 4th grade class we studied the subject of "India," and I decided to imitate the pictures of yogis standing on their heads with their legs folded in Lotus pose (*Padmāsana*)[2].

Many years later, after starting to study Iyengar yoga, I always had a *Sirsāsana* rope hanging somewhere in my house. My children were always attracted to it, and when hanging topsy-turvy from the rope, my eldest daughter expressed her delight by saying: "it makes life fun!" – I think this describes the essence of inverted poses: they make life so much better! Today I cannot imagine my life without them.

No doubt, inverted poses are the hallmark of yoga and its greatest gift to humanity. They, more than any other family of *āsana-s*, have deep effects on the mind. Our Guruji, B.K.S. Iyengar, used to practice inverted poses daily, staying in each pose 20 minutes or more. He continued through to the age of 95 – probably this had helped keep his mind so sharp and agile until his last day. Referring to the inverted poses, Geeta Iyengar expresses the importance of these *āsana-s* in the following words:

"The āsana-s belonging to these groups will take care of general health such as postural and functional correction of the body. They will take care of circulation, digestion, excretion and so on. You often avoid the practice of Śīrṣāsana and Sarvāngāsana, whereas it is Śīrṣāsana, along with the variations… and Sarvāngāsana, with the variations… which are very important in order to keep hormonal balance. Just as we take a bath everyday, we eat food, drink water and sleep at night, similarly we have to practise these āsana-s every day. We have to make it a habit to see that in our practice programme, even if nothing else is done, headstand, shoulder-stand and variations are always done. If you keep on with such a practice you will understand how much it is of help to maintain hormonal balance. It is only during menstruation that you should avoid Śīrṣāsana, Sarvāngāsana and other inversions."[3]

Inverted poses change the direction of gravity in the body and shift the bearing load to the arms, shoulders, chest and neck. They present a challenge for most students. In my experience, props can play an important role in introducing inversions gradually and safely until the student feels ready for the final poses. For all these reasons, I view the present volume as central to the *Props for Yoga* series.

Finally, I would like to take this opportunity to thank the many yoga practitioners who expressed interest in and commented on my previous books. Your enthusiasm has inspired me greatly. I hope to continue this project and cover additional families of *āsana-s* in future volumes.

Eyal Shifroni, February, 2017

[2] I still have a photo showing me in *Sirsāsana* while dressed with an Indian costume.

[3] From a transcript of the lecture: *Practice of women during the whole month* given by Geeta (emphases done by author)

Table of Contents

Chapter 4: Changing perspectives - Inverted Poses *(Viparīta Karaṇi Sthiti)* / 1

Detailed Table of Contents

Introduction

. . . .

N o t e : This Introduction is a slight modification of the Introduction to Volume II of this series. For the convenience of those who have already read the Introduction, I have indicated the sections that have been added or modified.

Yoga was revealed by the ancient sages as a way of spiritual realization and transformation; it was transmitted to us by a succession of sages *(rishis)* and Gurus. Texts like *The Yoga Sutras* of *Patañjali*, the *Bhagavad Gita* and the *Shiva Samhita* define and describe the essence of yoga, the yogic state, and yogic conduct. Many interpretations of these ancient texts have evolved over the years, including several books by my own teacher, *Yogācharya* B.K.S. Iyengar.

Yoga is not just a theory; it is a practical philosophy, a path to be travelled with intention, action, sensitivity and dedication. Only by putting the *sutras* into practice in our own lives can their full meaning and significance be revealed to us. Mere theoretical study of the texts will not lead to transformation and liberation. Guruji Iyengar's brilliant contribution has been in formulating ways in which the practice of *āsana* and *Prānāyāma* can be used to transform our bodies and minds through self-reflection, seeking to achieve the yogic state of knowing the eternal soul within.

Āsana-s are not mere exercises; they enable us to study our bodies and minds and to get acquainted with our limitations, tendencies and potentialities. Guruji Iyengar has developed the practice of *āsana* to a level of art and science. In his book *The Tree of Yoga*, he writes:

"Mahatma Gandhi did not practice all the aspects of yoga. He only followed two of its principles – non-violence and truth, yet through these two aspects of yoga, he mastered his own nature and gained independence for India. If part of yama could make Mahatma Gandhi so great, so pure, so honest and so divine, should it not be possible to take another limb of yoga – āsana – and through it reach the highest level of spiritual development? Many of you may say that performing āsana is a physical discipline, but if you speak in this way without knowing the depth of āsana, you have already fallen from the grace of yoga."[1]

In that book, Guruji Iyengar shows how all the eight limbs of *Ashtānga* Yoga can be experienced through a deep practice and study of the third and fourth limbs (*āsana* and *Prānāyāma*). Practicing *āsana* as physical exercises has its own merit. It may keep your body flexible, healthy and light, but if you do not accompany your practice by observing and studying your mind, you will miss the opportunity to develop your intelligence and to uplift your consciousness (By 'intelligence' I do not refer merely to one's IQ level but rather to one's ability to perceive one's self and one's surroundings without biases; to act skillfully in the pursuit of good according to one's own values and sense of truth).

Looking at *āsana* practice in light of Guruji Iyengar's teachings, we can understand the role of yoga props in his method. It is because such props – a wide range of equipment and accessories that he invented to aid the practice – allow people of all age groups and health conditions to enjoy the gifts of yoga. Indeed, the introduction of props, together with Guruji Iyengar's detailed instructions and thorough interpretation of ancient yoga texts have enabled millions to realize his vision of "Yoga is for All."

About the Use of Props

· ·

This is how Guruji Iyengar explains why he introduced props into his practice and teaching:

"I was preoccupied trying various ways to improve and perfect my own practice. I used to pick up stones and bricks lying on the roads and used them as 'supports' and 'weight bearers' to make progress in my mastery of āsana…

*Props help to perform the āsana-s with ease… The student understands and learns āsana faster on props as the brain remains passive. Through passive brain one learns to be alert in body and mind. **Props are guides to self-learning**[5]. They help accurately without mistakes." (In: 70 Glorious years of Yogācharya B.K.S. Iyengar, page 391)*

[4] *The Tree of Yoga* in the chapter:

The depth of *āsana*

[5] Highlighted by present author

Christian Pisano adds to that:

"Props thus allow us to unfold the space of an āsana and acquaint us with certain āsana that may otherwise be too difficult to practice. Props create understanding of the correct gesture (mudra) and attitude (bhava) of āsana. Props let us stay longer in an āsana, thus permitting deeper penetration of unexplored bodily regions."[6]

While props are an important characteristic of Iyengar Yoga, they should not be confused with its essence. Props are a means for achieving an end - such as alignment, stability, precision, and prolonged stays in *āsana*.

The usage of props covered here is intended to direct awareness to different aspects of the *āsana* and to different parts of the body, in order to deepen and enhance the understanding of the *āsana*. At the same time, practitioners should be careful not to develop dependency on props; rather, props should be employed intelligently in pursuit of a mature and mindful practice of *āsana*.

Guruji Iyengar continues his description:

"Now, talking of the pros and cons of using props, one of the criticisms leveled against props is that one becomes habituated and lacks the will to attempt doing independently. Is this the fault of props? Certainly not! Props are to feel the āsana. But I never say that they should be used on a permanent basis. Props give the sense of direction. When sense of direction sets in, I want my pupils to do the āsana independently sooner or later... The props are meant to give a sense of direction, alignment and understanding of the āsana."

Ultimately the body and mind are also external props to help "the seer to dwell in his own true splendor" (*Yoga Sutras of Patañjali*, I.3), or as Pisano expresses it:

"... Props can be regarded as an outer weave that points to the very essence of the āsana, in a purely subjective way. There will therefore always be some swaying between using an external prop and using the body itself as a prop. Ultimately, the body-mind is itself only an external prop."

 There are many ways in which props can be used to enhance our understanding of *āsana-s*:

- When used for support props allow us to **stay longer in difficult *āsana-s*** with stability (*Sthirata*), spaciousness and quietness (*Sukhata*). For example, *Viparīta Dandāsana* is an advanced back bend; when we do it without support, most of us struggle, breathe heavily, get tired quickly. Doing the pose supported by a chair or a wooden arch, allows us to let go of the excessive effort and to experience inner space and quietness, or in *Patañjali*'s words, *Sthira Sukham*.

[6] *The Hero's Contemplation, p. 109*

- Props can be used to **make the pose more difficult**. For example, in *Adho Mukha Śvānāsana*, when a helper pushes a block against our buttocks he or she actually makes the pose more difficult (see Variation 7 of this pose on page 38 of Volume 1). But this push teaches our muscles to work in the right direction. The prop is used not for support but rather for activation. When later we do the pose without this resistance, we can still imagine it and activate the muscles in the same way.

- Props can also be used to **decrease load from body parts that tend to be over loaded and make other parts heavier and more stable**. This is when a prop is used to change the geometry of the pose. For example, in standing *āsana-s* the back leg should function like an anchor – it should be heavy and stable. But often, when entering the pose, weight shifts to the front leg and the back leg loses its stability. Lifting the front leg on a chair or block (see Variation 10 of *Utthita Trikonāsana* on page 77 of Volume 1) changes the 'normal' geometry of the pose and thus allows us to feel how a well performed pose should be.

- Still other uses of props have **only mental effects**. For example, placing a belt under the outer foot of the back leg in *Utthita Trikonāsana* (as in Variation 3 of this pose on page 70 of Volume 1) does not support the pose and does not make it more difficult. Neither it changes the geometry of the pose – the whole purpose of this usage is to bring sensation and awareness to a body part.

To sum it up, props make it possible for every person to enhance his/her *Sādhanā* (study and discipline of yoga), regardless of physical limitations. By using props adequately one can:

- Perform *āsana-s* which are difficult to perform independently
- Achieve and maintain correct alignment during the practice
- Stay longer and relax in challenging *āsana-s*, thus attaining their full benefit
- Study and investigate *āsana-s* on a deeper level
- Continue practicing and improve her/his health condition even while suffering from chronic or temporary limitations and injuries.

The props used in this book

  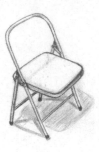

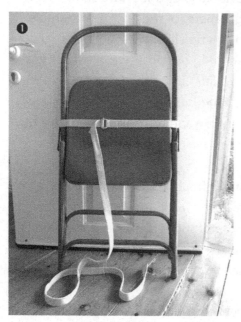

Looping around the chair to prevent unfolding

There are many props available, some are standard, and others are special and sophisticated. In this book I limit myself almost entirely to standard, widely available props. These are:

- blankets
- bolsters
- blocks – wooden, cork and rubber
- flat foam blocks
- belts – normal size and long
- ropes
- folded chairs
- wall – also wall corner

In a few places I present usage of wall or ceiling hooks and occasionally some simple special props. All these props are not expensive and can be easily stored and used at home.

The photos show the props I have in my center, which are largely compatible with those used in RIMYI (Pune). If you have props with different sizes (e.g., thicker blankets, or wider blocks) then you will have to adjust accordingly.

Just a few notes about the usage of chairs:

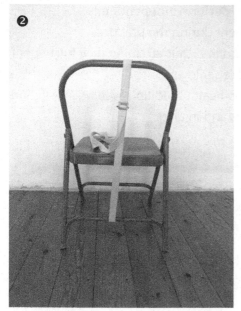

Looping around the backrest and back rung to prevent folding

- In many poses it is advisable to place a sticky mat on the seat of the chair. You do not need a full-size mat for this – a piece of about 40 cm × 40 cm (16 inches × 16 inches) is enough. It is handy to have a few pieces like this; so whenever a sticky mat becomes worn out, cut it and keep the pieces for future use.

- In some cases we want to use the chair when it is folded. To prevent it from unfolding, tie a belt as shown in ❶.

- In other cases we want to prevent the chair from folding. For this tie the chair as shown in ❷.

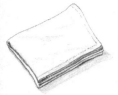 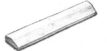 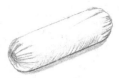

How not to use props

· ·

This series of *Props for Yoga* is written out of a strong belief that props can be a "guide to self-learning" and that they have an important role in exploring the *āsana-s* to a greater depth. However, if props are used because of laziness or lack of determination, to pamper one in her or his practice, then it is a wrong usage. It is tempting to rely on props and to avoid the effort (*Tapas*) needed to make progress. However, one should not only look for comfort in the *āsana-s*; the actions that should be done can only be learnt by *Abhyāsa* – repetitive, persistent and continuous effort (*sutra* I.14). Using props to avoid this effort will weaken your *Sādhanā* and stop your progress. The right approach is to use props in order to learn a specific action or a specific effect and then attempt to recreate that effect and/or action when doing the classic *āsana* without props.

Restorative poses have an important role in the overall balance of one's practice. However, if you are able to practice actively and choose to practice restoratively too often, then you foster stagnation and inertia (*Tamas*) instead of interest and dynamism.

About this Guide

The *Props for Yoga* series is the fruit of my nearly 40 years of Yoga *Sādhanā*. In the course of these rewarding years of daily practice and study, every day brings with it a new feeling, a new observation, a new insight. This book has evolved from this continuous journey of practice and study, be it in my own studio; at RIMYI, under Guruji, Geeta and Prashant Iyengar; in countless workshops that I took or gave in Israel and around the world; and last but not least – from the daily work with teachers and students at my own Iyengar Yoga Center in Israel.

Often, when preparing a class or a workshop, I search for new ways of highlighting the principles of *āsana* practice using props. I believe that many of my colleagues share a similar need. *Props for Yoga* is my modest attempt to address this need.

Since the original publication of *Light on Yoga*, the book which laid the foundation of the 'Iyengar Method', many books have been written in an attempt to elaborate and explain the wealth of knowledge embedded in that fundamental and by now classic text. The most prominent one is the beautiful book by Guruji Iyengar himself: *Yoga – the Path to Holistic Health*. Geeta's book: *A Gem for Women* and her booklets: *Yoga in Action, Preliminary and Intermediate-I courses* are important additions to that body of knowledge. Other books like *Yoga the Iyengar Way* by Silva, Mira & Shyam Mehta further clarify and specify the method. Most of these books, however, are intended for the general public, and cover mostly the basic usage of props. There are also several books showing the use of props specifically for Yoga Therapy. The present guide is intended primarily for teachers and experienced practitioners of the Iyengar Yoga method. It presents and explores a much greater variety of ways to use props. While some of the variations may be well known, many others are new and innovative ways that have not been documented yet.

My first book, *A Chair for Yoga*, focused on the use of a single prop in the practice of a wide variety of *āsana-s*. In contrast, each volume of the *Props for Yoga* series focuses on one or two family of *āsana-s*, but utilizes a variety of prop types. I purposefully limit the discussion to the simple, most commonly available props such as blocks, belts, blankets, walls, bolsters, ropes, etc.

The present book is the third in the series. Volume I focused on standing *āsana-s*, while Volume II covers sitting *āsana-s* and forward extensions. This Volume III covers the main inverted *āsana-s*, and contains four practice sequences which incorporate these *āsana-s* (see Appendix 3.1).

The Structure of the Guide

For each *āsana* a number of variations with different props are offered. Each variation is presented in the following order:

a. Props in use
b. Short introduction
c. Step-by-Step Instructions
d. Effects of practicing this variation
e. Tips – special points to observe in this variation
f. Applicability – in what other *āsana-s* the prop can be used in this way

Illustrated by photos, the **Step-by-Step Instructions** (part c), provide the technical information on how to position the body and use the props. The **Effects** section explains the desired effects of using the props in the specified manner and what can be learnt from it. The **Tips** section gives some clues regarding physical and mental actions you should do while staying in the *āsana* in order to get the desired effects.

N o t e :   *Āsana* practice works on many levels. Our presentation refers mostly to the seen and explicit level, the *annamayakośa* (the structural, anatomic body). However, *āsana-s* also affect the more internal *kośa-s* including the organic-physiological sheath (*pranamayakośa*) and the psychological sheath (*manomayakośa*). This text, being a practical guide, focuses on the technical aspects of the practice. This does not mean that the deeper effects of the practice are less important. I invite you – the reader - to pursue and experience these internal effects on your own.

How to
Use this Guide

Keep the following in mind when using this guide:

- This Guide is not a substitute for learning with a certified Iyengar Yoga teacher. The subtleties of the instructions in the Iyengar Yoga method cannot adequately be captured in a book. So, while it can help you study and explore the *āsana-s*, please remember that no guide can observe you and correct mistakes you may perform while doing a variation.

- This Guide does not provide instructions for therapeutic usages of props. People who wish to adopt yoga as a therapy treatment should consult a teacher who is certified to deal with their case[7].

- Work by comparison and analysis: Do the pose several times with and without the props. Observe your sensations when doing the pose with the prop and then try to recreate those sensations without the prop. Do not use the props habitually, but rather use them for learning in a creative and innovative way; study and compare the effects to enhance your understanding. Do not develop dependency on props; rather, employ them mindfully. Always remain fresh and alert!

- The possibilities are virtually endless; use your imagination and creativity to find new ways of using props.

You should also note the following:

1. For the sake of clarity, each of the presented variations focuses on the use of a single prop, or on one specific way to work in an *āsana*. However, some of the variations can be practiced in combination or in sequence. To avoid confusion, I do not show such combinations, but rather encourage you to try them on your own.

2. To facilitate quick access to the material in the guide, use the detailed Index and the Table of Contents. The Index contains references to the variations according to the prop used and the *āsana* taken and the prop used.

[7] For therapeutic uses of props,
see the books of Lois Steinberg at:
www.loissteinberg.com/booksaudio/

3. When working in pairs, it is recommended to work with a partner of the same gender and, as much as possible, of the same size and flexibility. Always be watchful and prudent when helping other people.

4. Certain variations refer to plates in *Light on Yoga*. Those are marked by the symbol LOY followed by the plate number. For example, "LOY Pl. 100" refers to plate number 100 in *Light on Yoga*.

CAUTION

 Users of this guide must have a solid foundation in yoga practice, preferably obtained through regular classes with a certified Iyengar Yoga teacher. Some of the variations shown in this guide are advanced and should not be attempted without guidance and supervision. The author takes no responsibility for any injury or damage that may occur due to improper use of the material presented.

Enjoy your practice!

. . . .

If you have any comments or feedback…I'd love to hear it.
Please write to me at:
eyal@theiyengaryoga.com

Chapter 4
Changing perspectives – Inverted Poses
(Viparīta Karaṇi Sthiti)

About the Inverted Poses

"Whatever nectar flows from the moon which is divine form, it is all swallowed up by the sun. Hence the body decays."

"There exists a divine process by which the sun is duped…"

"If one's navel is high and palate is low, then the sun in above and the moon below. This position, the inverted pose (Viparīta Karaṇi), is to be learned through the instructions of a Guru."

Hatha Yoga Pradīpika III, 77-79

The above quote from *Hatha Yoga Pradīpika* describes symbolically the extraordinary benefits of the inverted poses. The downward flow of the nectar which is swallowed up by the sun, causes the body to decay. Inverted poses reverse, or at least slow this process. Indeed, the inverted poses – the unique gift of yoga - are a great boon. These poses take us on an inner journey into the core of our being. They touch and heal us at a deep level; they penetrate deep within, where our fears are hidden yet also where our powers and joys can be found.

Geeta Iyengar and Lois Steinberg describe the physiological and mental benefits of inversions in the following words[8]:

"… In addition to the reproductive effects, inversions also benefit the endocrine, lymphatic, circulatory, digestive, respiratory, urinary, excretory and central nervous systems. The pituitary, pineal, thyroid and adrenal glands receive a proper blood supply. Inversions are the greatest poses for balancing hormones which are also connected to maintaining bone density. Constipation, flatulence, and hemorrhoids are alleviated. The urinary tract, urethra, kidneys and bladder benefit from the relief given by the anti-gravitational force. Again, mineral loss from the bones is checked when the muscles and bones are going against gravity. The resilience of the lungs is improved, and the body is kept warm. Retention of fluid, edema of the lower legs is reduced. The brain receives a healthy current of blood, is rejuvenated, and clarity of thoughts predominates. Sleep problems may improve. A state of equilibrium, balance, and health is established with regular practice of inversion."

[8] *Woman's Yoga Practice* by Geeta Iyengar and Lois Steinberg, p. 120

Inverted poses are the gateway to *Prānāyāma* practice; they teach us what a yogic mind is – alert, passive, neutral and non-reactive. Inversions are very central in the Iyengar Yoga method and long stays in *Sirsāsana* and *Sarvāngāsana* are part and parcel of the daily routine of every serious practitioner. Guruji Iyengar summarized his description of the effects of *Sirsāsana* in *Light on Yoga*, with these inspirational words:

"Regular and precise practice of Sirsāsana develops the body, disciplines the mind and widens the horizons of the spirit. One becomes balanced and self-reliant in pain and pleasure, loss and gain, shame and fame and defeat and victory."

I strongly identify with the following words of Geeta Iyengar and Lois Steinberg [9]:

"The benefits of Sirsāsana and Sarvāngāsana cannot be over emphasized. Practitioners of inverted postures experience the effects daily. If circumstances truncate the time for practice, they know to do Sirsāsana and Sarvāngāsana as their benefits would be missed."

These two key inversions complement each other; *Sirsāsana* is dynamic and active, it is a sun (*Surya*) pose, whereas *Sarvāngāsana* is quieting and contemplative; it is a moon (*Chandra*) pose. My feeling is that *Sirsāsana* sharpens the eyes while *Sarvāngāsana* opens and nourishes the ears. In *Sirsāsana* one looks forward at eye level seeing the surrounding from a new and unfamiliar angle; this stimulates the eyes. *Sarvāngāsana* creates space in the inner ears and increases the circulation in that region. The eyes become less functional in *Sarvāngāsana* and its cycle, and often one tends to close them. Vision is more external than the auditory sense. Guruji Iyengar considered the eyes as being connected to the brain and the ears as being connected to the mind; this further explains the alert passivity of *Sirsāsana*, compared with the inwardness induced by *Sarvāngāsana*. Seeing draws us to the outer world while hearing encourages attention for our inner space; this is probably why most meditation practices are done with closed eyes. The *Ākasha* (space) element is connected with sound. Hence *Sarvāngāsana* draws the mind inward more than *Sirsāsana*.

In a talk given on the occasion of Guruji Iyengar's 79th Birthday celebration, he characterized the inverted *āsana-s* as follows [10]:

"One cannot do Sirsāsana without using the head and one cannot do Setu Bandha Sarvāngāsana without using the heart. Each āsana has its own characteristic and as such we have to observe and study from where the source of action takes place… In Setu Bandha Sarvāngāsana and Halāsana the brain remains silent but the seat of the heart remains attentive, while in Sirsāsana the brain is attentive while the seat of the heart remains pensive."

[9] *Woman's Yoga Practice*

[10] *Astadala Yoga Mala, Vol. 8 p. 23*

Christian Pisano mentions the differences in the effects of these poses on the *Bandhas*:

"Sirsāsana unfolds two diaphragms or hearts. It is a very important āsana for understanding the suction and spreading of the pelvic floor, which is the heart of Mūlabandha, and the suction and spreading of the abdomen for Uddīyānabandha. The variations in Sirsāsana intensify this action. Sarvāngāsana and Halāsana pacify the vocal diaphragm and allow it to spread, whilst unblocking the neck and thus allowing Jālandharabandha to be unfolded. Setu Bandha Sarvāngāsana awakens all three bandhas.

Working with support is essential to this approach, firstly to cleanse certain regions and then to unfold the different colorations of breath into them. Hence, rope Sirsāsana, Viparīta Dandāsana on a chair or bench, Sarvāngāsana on a chair, half Halāsana with supported thighs, Setu Bandha Sarvāngāsana on a bench and Viparīta Karaṇi all become precious instruments for contemplating the different modalities of breath."[11]

And indeed, in *Sirsāsana* the respiratory diaphragm has more freedom of movement and the breathing tends to be *Samanic* (of the diaphragm and lower chest). In well-done *Sarvāngāsana*, on the other hand, the upper chest opens and breathing tends to be more *Prāṇic* and *Udanic* (central and top chest). To get this effect we need to use a platform to elevate the shoulders and upper arms above the head level – this also prevents undue pressure on the cervical vertebrae and is considered a must in the Iyengar Yoga method. I explore many options of using a platform in the section on *Sarvāngāsana*.

For the above characterizations, it is clear why *Sarvāngāsana* and its cycle appear usually toward the end of the practice sequence, and certainly after *Sirsāsana* and its cycle. It is recommended to stay in the *Sarvāngāsana* cycle one and a half times longer than in the *Sirsāsana* cycle.

The duration of staying in inversions is a key factor. To get their full anatomical, physiological, mental, psychological and spiritual benefits, one needs to stay in them for more than just a few minutes. The internal processes that take place need time to yield effects. As Prashant Iyengar terms it: "you can't put rice in boiling water and expect it to be ready after just one minute." In the same way, going up to *Sirsāsana* just to get down after a minute or so, is all right for a beginner, but has limited effects compared to staying in the *āsana* for 10 minutes or more. Every now and then I dedicate a large portion of my practice to prolonged stays in inversions (up to 30 minutes in *Sirsāsana* and 45 minutes in *Sarvāngāsana & Halāsana*) – this is a very deep practice and it changes completely the state of the mind! Remember though that quality is more important than quantity – it is better to stay 5 minutes with full attention and awareness than to struggle to extend the time when the pose does not feel right.

[11] *The Hero's contemplation*, by C.
Pisano, p. 124.

Staying for 10 minutes or more in *Sirsāsana* or *Sarvāngāsana* is challenging both physically and mentally. Being aware of that, Guruji Iyengar has invented props that allow almost everyone to savor the flavor of long stays in inversions. There are many props and arrangements of blankets, bolsters and blocks which help to extend the duration of the stay in these poses without excessive effort. This is true even for individuals who suffer from structural deformities in the cervical spine.

CAUTION Avoid practicing inversions if you suffer from:

- High blood pressure
- Eye or ear problems
- Heart disease
- Dizziness or nausea
- Women shouldn't do inversions during the menstruation days. See the section below for substitutes for menstruating women

If you suffer from **neck problems**, you can still practice inversions with props as described in some of the variations below, but do so under the guidance of an experienced Iyengar Yoga teacher.

Substitution for the inverted poses for women during menses

In the Iyengar Yoga method there is a lot of knowledge about women's practice during the monthly menstrual cycle. Books like: *The Woman's Yoga Book* by Bobby Clennell and *Geeta S. Iyengar's Guide to a Woman's Yoga Practice* by Lois Steinberg are excellent references that deal with the subject thoroughly. These books suggest special sequences which are beneficial during menses. Women should study these books and practice the sequences presented in them during menstruation. However, in many cases, menstruating women can keep attending their regular classes and inform the teacher about this, so she or he can suggest alternatives for the *āsana-s* which are contra indicated during menses. Inverted *āsana-s* obviously must be avoided[12]. The best substitution for *Sirsāsana* is a supported version of *Viparīta Dandāsana* (❶, ❷ & ❸), and for *Sarvāngāsana* is a supported version of *Setu Bandha Sarvāngāsana* (❹, ❺ & ❻)

In *Viparīta Dandāsana* the head is vertically inverted like in *Sirsāsana* and the pose has many of the energetic qualities of *Sirsāsana* – it is stimulating, alerting and induces sharpness combined with passivity. In *Setu Bandha Sarvāngāsana* the head is horizontal like in *Sarvāngāsana* and this is relaxing, quieting and induces inwardness and humbleness much like *Sarvāngāsana*.

[12] The reasons for that are explained in the above books as well as in many of Geeta Iyengar's writings.

The following photos show how to adapt these back-bends to menstruation. Note that the legs are supported to avoid over stretching of the abdominal organs and the chest is supported to create opening, so the breath can flow softly and deeply. The lengthening and widening of the pelvic region alleviate menstrual cramps. The poses provide deep rest combined with stimulation of the brain created by the increased circulation to the head region.

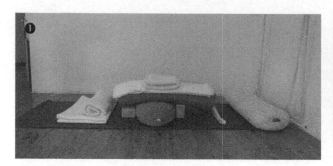

Props arrangement for *Viparīta Dandāsana*

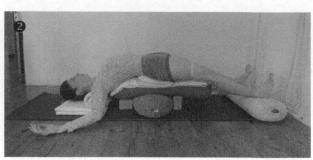

Viparīta Dandāsana on cross bolsters

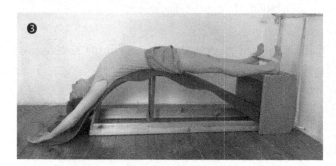

Viparīta Dandāsana on a back bender

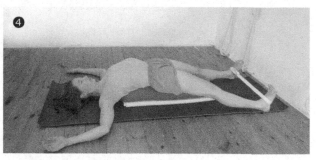

Setu Bandha Sarvāngāsana on a lengthwise bolster

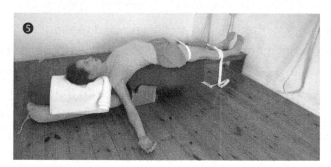

Setu Bandha Sarvāngāsana on a bench and *Viparīta Karaṇi* box

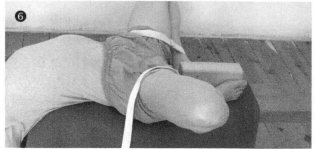

Setu Bandha Sarvāngāsana on a bench – *Baddha Koṇāsana* variation

Sālamba Sirsāsana I

Donald Moyer characterizes *Sirsāsana* beautifully in his book[13]:

> "Traditionally, Sālamba Sarvāngāsana was considered as the mother of all poses because of its nurturing quality, and Sālamba Sirsāsana as the father of all poses because of its clarifying effect. Initially, Sālamba Sirsāsana is a challenging pose that requires strength in your shoulders and flexibility in your shoulders to avoid compression in your neck, as well as strength in your lower back and abdomen to support the weight of your legs. Ultimately, however, you will discover the place of inner balance in the pose, where your mind is clear and alert, your body calm and suspended, and your whole being poised between action and reflection."

Christian Pisano writes[14]:

> "Inverted āsana, even Sirsāsana, which is a stimulating āsana, teach the art of resorption. It is in these āsana that the withdrawal of all the energies into their source culminates."

[13] *Yoga – awakening the inner body*, Donald Moyer, p. 37

[14] *The Hero's contemplation*, p. 94

Sirsāsana Basics

In order to enjoy *Sirsāsana* you need strong arms and upper back and sufficient movement in the shoulder region. To prepare for *Sirsāsana* practice all the basic standing *āsana-s*, as well as *Adho Mukha Śvānāsana* and *Adho Mukha Vṛkṣāsana* (full arm balance). The forearms and hands are the base of the pose; the entire forearms should be pressed to the floor and the upper arms should be lifted. I start with variations that help learning the basics of the pose.

Sālamba Sirsāsana I

Variation 1
Preparing the base of the pose:
Activating the arms and shoulders

Effects

This preparation teaches the correct base for the pose: the placement of the forearms, fingers and head. The resistance of the wall helps to mobilize and lift the shoulders. Practice this variation to strengthen the arms, shoulders and upper back muscles and to create movement in the shoulders region. It is crucial to repeat this until these muscles are strong enough and it is possible to keep the shoulder girdle stable while moving the pelvis up and toward the wall. Do not attempt Sirsāsana before this is achieved.

Props
wall

This preparation is called *Ardha Sirsāsana* (see also: *Yoga in Action, Preliminary course*, P. 81).

→ Kneel next to the wall and place both elbows in line and shoulder-width apart.

T i p s

✔ Use the edge of the mat to ensure that the elbows are in line.

❯ Extend the forearms forward and place them with palms facing upward ❶.

❯ Rub the skin of the forearms on the mat as you turn the forearms such that the outer forearms (ulna bones), outer palms and little fingers are pressing the mat.

❯ Interlock the fingers such that no space is left in between them. Move forward until the knuckles touch the wall. Round the wrists to form a cup-shaped palms.

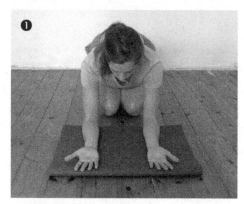
Placing the forearms for *Sirsāsana*

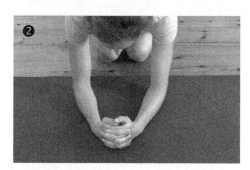
Interlocking the fingers

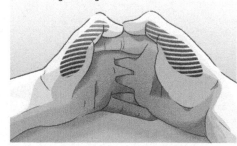
Figure 1 The portion of the thumbs that touch the head

❯ Align the fingers parallel to the floor, each fingertip rests in between the bones of the roots of the two corresponding fingers of the other hand.

❯ To ensure tight interlock, move the right index finger to the left and the left index finger to the right. Place the thumbs one on top of the other or one tip against the other ❷.

❯ Cross also the little fingers and extend the outer hands (little fingers side) away from the head.

❯ Place the crown (top) of the head on the mat and move it well into the cup-shaped palms (see "Finding the crown of the head" below). Support the back of the head by the roots of the thumbs. Figure 1 shows the regions of the palms that touch the head.

Sālamba Sirsāsana I

Variation 1 (Cont'd)
Preparing the base of the pose:
Activating the arms and shoulders

> Press the forearms down to lift the shoulders. Move the shoulders away from the ears and neck, both upward and sideways. Move the shoulder blades in (away from the wall) and stabilize the shoulder girdle.

> Straighten the knees and slowly step forward toward the wall. As you do so, push the knuckles against the wall, move the shoulders up and away from the wall and make the upper back concave.

> Tighten the quadriceps to lift the thighs and buttocks. Stretch your spine and, pushing with your feet, bring the pelvis closer to the wall without rounding the upper back – keep it concave and move it away from the wall ❸.

> Stay in this position from 30 to 45 sec., then rest and repeat a few times.

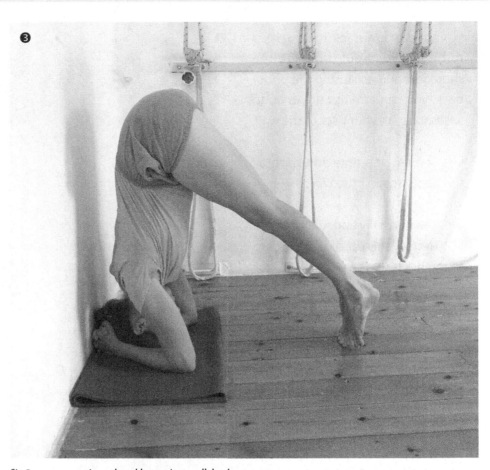

❸

Sirsāsana preparation – knuckles against wall, back concave

T i p s
✔ Look at your elbows to make sure that each outer elbow is placed in line with the corresponding outer shoulder.

✔ Interlock the fingers well to form a cup-shape structure, but do not tense the fingers or the palms.

✔ The fingers should be parallel to the floor. When going up to *Sirsāsana* do not let the index fingers spread, as this will weaken the base of the pose.

✔ To develop the arms symmetrically, alternate the finger-interlock between *Sirsāsana* practices.

Variation 1 (Cont'd)
Preparing the base of the pose:
Activating the arms and shoulders

Sirsāsana with the back to the wall

→ When you are able to step closer to the wall without dropping the shoulders and collapsing the upper back, you can attempt going up to *Sirsāsana* with your back to the wall:

> Lift one leg at a time and support the heels against the wall.

> Breathe normally and relax! Stretch both legs evenly up, sliding the back of the heels up the wall.

> Keep lifting the shoulders.

> Keeping the back of the head and the lumbar close to the wall, move the shoulder blades, buttocks and tailbone away from the wall ❶.

> Stay for a minute or two and then go down leg by leg. Stay in *Adho Mukha Vīrāsana* for at least 30 seconds before lifting the head.

If everything is okay, you can learn to balance without the wall:

> Move one heel away from the wall and stretch the corresponding leg upward while pressing the other heel to the wall. Then repeat on the other leg ❸.

> Move the other heel away from the wall and stretch both legs upward for independent *Sirsāsana* ❹.

> Go down leg after leg.

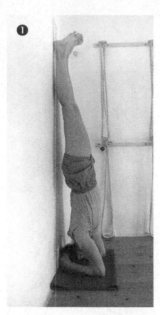

❶

Sirsāsana heels on the wall

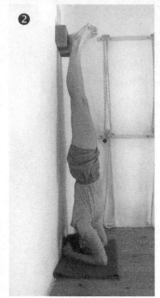

❷

Learning the verticality of *Sirsāsana*

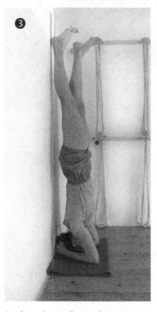

❸

Back to the wall, one leg away

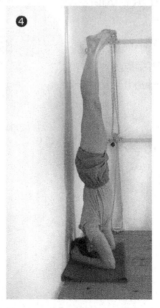

❹

Moving from the wall to independent *Sirsāsana*

T i p s

✔ It is recommended to have the first experience of *Sirsāsana* in the middle of the room with the help of a teacher. This prevents the student from developing dependence upon the wall. Use the wall for balance only after that first experience.

✔ The back of the heels and back of the head should be in one vertical line; therefore, you need to keep the head as close as possible to the wall.

✔ To get a vertical pose, ask a friend to place a rubber or foam block between your heels and the wall as shown in ❷.

✔ Try to sense if your legs are not slanting left or right. Ask a teacher or a friend to observe and verify that your head and legs are centered.

Sālamba Sirsāsana I

Variation 1 (Cont'd)
Preparing the base of the pose:
Activating the arms and shoulders

Moving the upper back and the buttocks in

⟶ A crucial action in *Sirsāsana* is to move the shoulder blades, thoracic dorsal spine and the buttocks forward (into the body). The wall can be used to learn these actions.

❯ Instead of placing the head close to the wall, place it at about 8-10 cm (3-4 inches) away from the wall.

❯ Go up to *Sirsāsana* with your back to the wall and place the heels on the wall ❶.

❯ Push the heels against the wall and use this to lift the shoulder blades and to move them, as well as the thoracic dorsal spine, away from the wall.

❯ Move also the buttocks away from the wall and lift the top buttocks toward the heels as you slide the heels up the wall ❷.

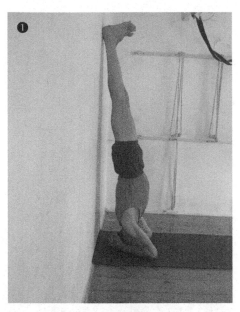

Sirsāsana slightly away from the wall

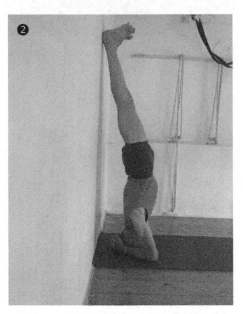

Using the wall to move the upper back and the buttocks in

T i p s

✓ Keep the big toes joined to sensitize the feet and let the energy flow from the head upward to the toes.

✓ As long as there is no pressure on the neck, you can stay in the pose safely. If, after staying for some time, your arms get tired and you cannot lift the shoulders anymore, do not stay in the pose: Come down, rest, and then try again.

✓ However, do not go up and down more than 2-3 times in a row, as this may disturb the nervous system.

Sālamba Sirsāsana I

Variation 2
Finding the crown of the head

Effects
Several methods are given to find the position of the crown (top) of the head.
This is essential for correct Sirsāsana.

Props
1-2 blocks

Students often ask where exactly the crown or top of the head is located. In my experience, the best way to clarify this is to use a block in order to sensitize this region:

→ Sit or stand upright. Make sure that the spine, neck and head are on one vertical line.

❯ Place a block horizontally on the top of the head and balance it.

❯ The region of the head that touches the block is the crown (top) of the head. This region should touch the floor when doing *Sirsāsana*.

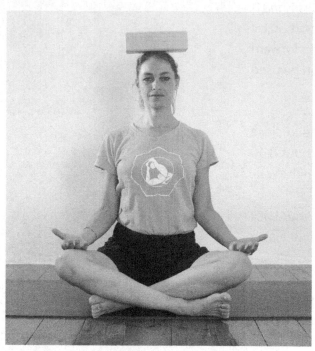

Using a block to sensitize the crown (top) of the head

T i p s

For beginners, it is acceptable to place the head slightly toward the forehead, as this helps to maintain the natural curvature of the neck, and hence to keep it soft. But, in order to get the full benefits of the pose the head should be absolutely vertical. In this way, the back and front parts of the brain are aligned and receive even circulation and stimulation. This gives a feeling of poise and harmony. Advanced practitioners should therefore learn to stand on the very top of the head.

You can also study the vertical position of the head in *Uttānāsana* with head support or in *Prasārita Padottānāsana*.

→ Depending of the height of the head in your *Uttānāsana*, place in front of you a block or two (usually one lying flat on the top of the other).

❯ Stand with legs slightly apart and bend down to *Uttānāsana*.

❯ Place the tips of the thumbs inside the ears and the fingers on the occiput. Roll the inner ears forward and release the back of the neck until you feel that the ears are vertical ❶.

❯ Look in between the legs, parallel to the floor.

❯ Then place the hands down and stay to sense the crown of the head ❷.

❯ You can do the same in *Prasārita Padottānāsana* with the top of the head on the floor ❸ or, if needed, on a block (not shown).

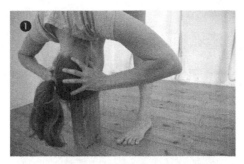

Uttānāsana with head support, using the fingers to roll the head

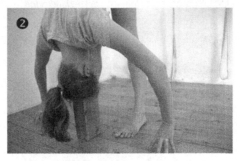

Uttānāsana with head support

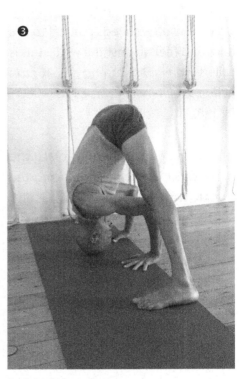

Prasārita Padottānāsana

Guruji Iyengar referred to the placement of the head in a talk[15]:

"When you rest on the crown of your head, do you know what the crown of the head is? Often while doing Sirsāsana resting on the head, people are aware only of the front part of the head and the balance of the body and not of the crown of the head and therefore the intellectual awareness touches the frontal body while the back of the body remains in the state of insensitivity... This single connecting thread from the head to the arches of the feet is the intelligence. The two heads – the crown of the head and the middle of the arches of the feet – are like the South pole and the North pole. They have to be evenly balanced in Sirsāsana. This is the spiritual or mystical root of Sirsāsana.'

T i p s

✔ When doing *Uttānāsana* or *Prasārita Padottānāsana* with head support, the load on the head is minimal, so you can easily roll the head back and forth to experiment various positions in order to develop the sensitivity to the effects of the angle of the head.

[15] *Astadala Yoga Mala*, Vol. 5, p. 236

Sālamba Sirsāsana I

Variation 3
Sirsāsana preparation: Feet against the wall

Effects
The feet support helps to lift the shoulders and to make the upper back concave.

Props
wall

In this Variation, Sirsāsana is done facing a wall, with legs parallel to the floor and feet against the wall – this is called Ūrdhva Dandāsana (see: Yoga in Action, Preliminary course, P. 83 & LOY Pl. 188).

→ First find where to place the head: Sit in Dandāsana facing the wall, with your feet against it and place the fingers in line with the buttocks. Mark that spot ❶.

❯ Place the crown of the head on the mat in the position marked by your fingers (which is where the buttocks were in Dandāsana).

❯ Place the forearms and elbows to form an isosceles triangle, as explained in the previous variation.

❯ Now climb up the wall until your legs are parallel to the floor ❷.

❯ Lift the front thighs and pelvis.

❯ Pushing against the wall, lift the shoulders, move the shoulder blades in (toward the wall) and make the upper back concave.

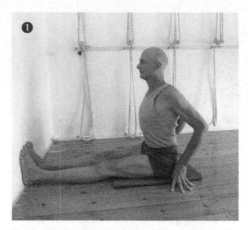

Finding the distance from the wall in Dandāsana

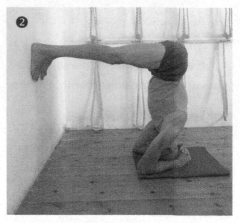

Ūrdhva Dandāsana - feet against wall

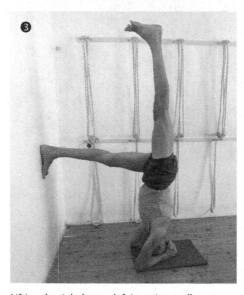

Lifting the right leg up, left is against wall

To learn to do the pose away from the wall:

❯ From Ūrdhva Dandāsana, lift the right leg and stretch it vertically up ❸.

❯ Without dropping the shoulders, lower the right leg and lift the left leg.

❯ Repeat until you feel stable. Now lift one leg and then the other: you are doing Sirsāsana with no wall behind you!

A note for the teacher:

🔖 This is an excellent way to help students overcome the dependency on the wall. Stand behind the student, support her/him and allow the student to find her/his own balance. From my experience, after two or three attempts when facing the wall, the student will be ready to stand on her/his own in the center of the room.

Overcoming the 'wall complex'

Many students, including long-time practitioners, do Sirsāsana only when there is a wall behind them, and feel insecure to do it away from the wall. Having a wall behind gives reassurance. Doing the pose facing the wall is a good way to build confidence for the independent pose. It enables one to experience the feeling of having no support behind the back, while leaving an option to lower one leg to the wall if shakiness or fear occurs.

Verifying the Correct Alignment of the Pose

Yoga is an inward journey, and in the *āsana-s* we have to gradually develop awareness that will allow us to know how exactly the body is positioned, without using external means.

In *Sirsāsana* especially, one does not see his/her own body so it is challenging to verify its correct alignment. Yet, this is crucial, since a crooked head or misaligned shoulders may cause injury. Until the awareness is developed one needs to use external means.

You can use a wall corner to measure yourself in the pose (as in the following Variations). When doing *Sirsāsana* away from a wall you can ask your teacher to check your alignment. When practicing at home, you can use a mirror. The mirror should extend all the way to the floor, so you can observe the head and arms. In my experience, even in a class situation a mirror can be sometimes helpful, since students who have a habitual asymmetry find it hard to correct their pose, unless they see the misalignment with their own eyes. However, do not develop dependency on the mirror, and learn to sense your alignment without relying on external means.

If a mirror is not available ask a friend to take photos of your pose from several angles. Study these photos, and if possible, also show them to your teacher, to get a better feedback.

> *"Your awareness and intelligence in head balance should produce a straight line on your body from your head to your heels. The inner intelligence should be parallel to the back body, the front body and the side body."* B.K.S. Iyengar[16]

Interestingly, in Hebrew the words 'awareness' and 'knowing' are derived from the same root.

[16] *Astadala Yoga Mala, Vol. 5, P. 80*

Effects

Finding the correct alignment is essential for extended relaxed stay in Sirsāsana. This Variation explains the correct alignment observing from the front, back and sides.

Checking the alignment from the front

Observing the pose from the front ❶ check the following points:

• Both elbows are on the same line and are equidistant from the midline of the body (a) (see also *Astadala Yoga Mala*: Vol. 8 Plate n. 20 & Vol. 7 Plate n. 49) the outer elbows are aligned with the outer shoulders (b)

• The midline of the body is vertical and centered, i.e., the centers of the: head, chest and pelvis and the meeting point of the big toes form a vertical line (not tilting left or right), which divides the body into two symmetrical halves (c)

• Both sides of the body are lifted evenly. Check the height of the eyes, shoulders, the corners of the pelvis and the feet (d) (see also Plate n. 47 in *Astadala Yoga Mala* Vol. 5)

• The body is not twisted left or right. Check that the nose is facing exactly forward (not turning left or right) and that the two nipples, the corners of the pelvis and the feet are aligned

• The centers of the legs and knees are facing forward, not projecting out (e). The toes are facing forward and the big toes are joined.

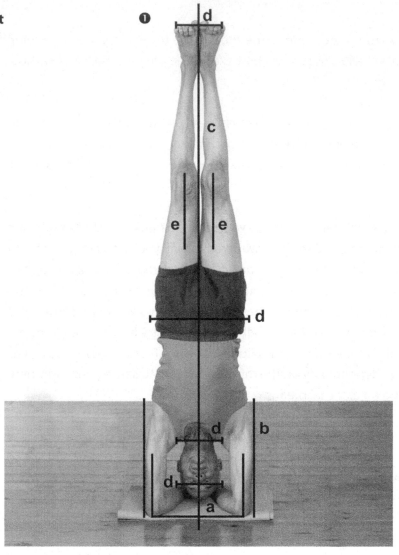

Checking left to right symmetry in *Sirsāsana*

Checking the alignment from the back ❷

Observing the pose from the back ❷ verify that:

- The midline of the body (center of the back of the head, tailbone and the meeting point of the heels) is vertical and the left and right sides are spread evenly (a)

- The distance between the shoulders and the ears is even on both sides and as large as in *Tadāsana* (see also Plates n. 24 & 49 in *Astadala Yoga Mala* Vol. 7) (b)

- Both shoulder blades are lifted and tucked in evenly (c)

- The buttocks are aligned and are not dropping toward the lumbar but are lifted toward the legs (d)

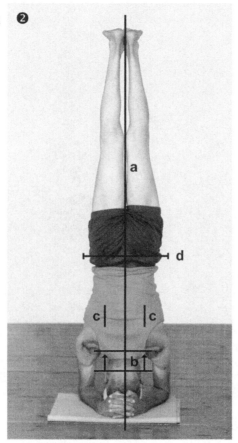

Alignment of *Sirsāsana* from the back

❸

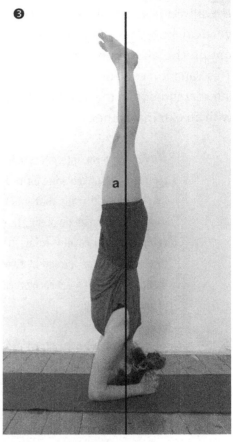

Alignment of *Sirsāsana* from the side

Checking the alignment from the side

Observing the pose from the side ❸ verify that:

- The center of the ear, shoulder joint, hip joint and ankle joint are all on the same vertical line (not slanting back or front) (a) (see also Plate n. 21 in *Astadala Yoga Mala* Vol. 4)

T i p s

✔ *When in Sirsāsana, feel the sides of the body. Stretch up from the outer armpits to the sides of the pelvis and from there to the outer ankles. This will help you to create and maintain the proper alignment of the pose..*

Sālamba Sirsāsana I

Variation 5
Verifying verticality: Using 'internal' wall corner

Effects
Non-symmetrical contact with the two walls forming the corner indicates that the pose is twisted or tilted. The walls provide support, guidance and safety, making this variation very useful in the learning stage.

Props
internal wall corner,
2 identical blocks

A wall corner provides a straight vertical line that can be used to gauge the alignment of *Sirsāsana*. This Variation explains how to use an internal corner, and the next one deals with an external corner.

> **Note:** The term 'internal corner' refers to the sunken edge formed by two vertical walls that meet each other at an angle of 90°. The term 'external corner' refers to the exposed edge formed by two vertical walls that meet each other at an angle of 270°.

→ Take two blocks and place them against the walls on each side. Interlock the fingers and place the cup shaped palms on the floor, all the way into the internal corner. Position the elbows against the blocks, equidistant from the two walls.

> Go up to *Sirsāsana* and place the buttocks and the heels symmetrically on the walls along the two sides of the corner.

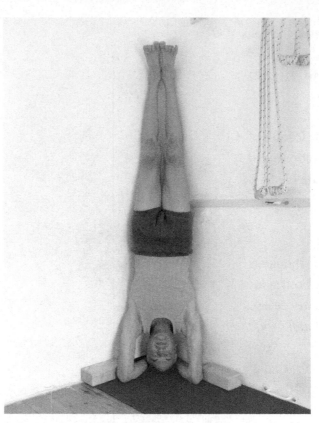

Sirsāsana with internal corner

> Slowly move the buttocks and the heels slightly away from the walls; stay for 30 to 60 seconds; then slowly move back to touch the walls. Check if both buttocks and both heels reach the walls at the same time.

> Experiment several times to find out if you have a consistent tendency to tilt the body or to get crooked. Observe and then correct according to the feedback you receive from the wall.

Sālamba Sirsāsana I

Variation 6
Verifying verticality: Using 'external' wall corner

The sharp edge of an external corner gives excellent feedback on the position of the head, spine and legs. It teaches both back-to-front and left-to-right (lateral) alignment, and enables one to check if there is a consistent tendency to tilt or twist the body while staying in the pose. Hence this is a very effective way to learn the alignment of Sirsāsana. Every practitioner can benefit from gauging herself/himself in this way from time to time.

Props
wall corner

Once you can balance in the middle of the room, you can use an external corner.

→ Instead of interlocking the fingers, press the palms against the walls on both sides of the corner.

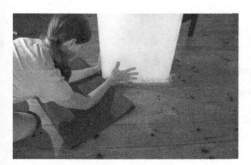

Placing the hands against external corner

> Place your elbows at shoulder width and go up to the pose.

> Position the middle of the occiput (the back of the skull), the tailbone and the meeting point of the heels on the corner.

> Keeping the back of the head and the heels on the vertical edge move the tailbone and the thoracic dorsal spine away from the corner. At the same time, move the lumbar spine towards the corner.

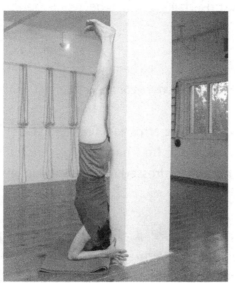

Sirsāsana with external corner

> After a while, move slightly away from the corner; stay for 30 to 60 seconds; then slowly move back to touch the corner. Check if both heels touch it concurrently and symmetrically. Observe how the vertebrae touch the corner.

> Experiment several times and see if you have a consistent tendency to tilt the body or to become crooked. Observe and then correct.

Tips

✔ Sharpen and elongate the spine by bringing its left side to the right and its right side to the left.

✔ Still another way to align yourself is to do the pose facing a vertical column, a wall or a window edge. Observing such a vertical line can help you check the verticality of the pose.

Arms and Shoulders

The arms and shoulders are the base of the pose; talking about the five elements, Guruji Iyengar said:

> *"What is the quality of the element 'earth'? It is heaviness… In Sirsāsana the forearms become the element of earth and the legs become the element of air… "[17]*

The first thing to learn therefore is how to use the arms as a firm and stable base for the pose. A question that is often asked is "how much weight should I bear on my head in *Sirsāsana*?". Guruji Iyengar addressed this question in an interview and said:

> *"If the hands are not protective, your shoulders collapse and the neck feels the weight. If you use the arms like the legs of tripod, you do not feel the weight of the body on your head or neck anymore. Do you feel the weight on your legs when you are walking? Similarly, when Sālamba Sirsāsana is done regularly, the doer feels no weight on the head. So, the secret of head balance is that you should not feel your body weight on your head and that is a perfect Sālamba Sirsāsana."[18]*

From my experience, there is no harm in bearing some weight on the head, as long as the neck is long and the back of the neck is soft. If however, you feel that your body weight is collapsing on the head and the vertebrae of the neck are compressed, then the pose is wrong. You must develop the ability to shift the body weight to the arms by activating the shoulders and shoulder blades correctly.

[17] *Astadala Yoga Mala, Vol. 6, p. 68-69*

[18] *Astadala Yoga Mala, Vol. 5, p. 81*

Sālamba Sirsāsana I

Variation 7
Stabilizing the arms: A belt on the elbows

Effects

The forearms and elbows are the foundation of Sirsāsana. If the elbows slip or shake, then the foundation becomes weak. In some cases, one elbow slips more than the other and the pose becomes uneven. This Variation keeps the elbows at the correct position. Working against the resistance of the belt activates and strengthens the arms and teaches to press the outer elbows down to the floor and to lift the inner arms up to the armpits.

Props

belt

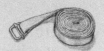

In *Sirsāsana* the outer elbows should be positioned exactly below the outer shoulders; using a belt one can verify this and keep the elbows in place.

→ Loop a belt around your elbows and tighten it to shoulder-width. Go up to *Sirsāsana*.

❯ Work the elbows against the resistance of the belt.

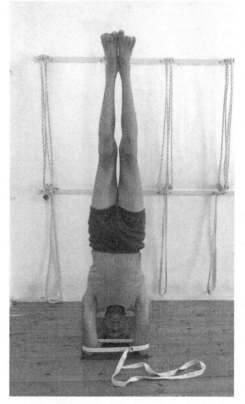

Sirsāsana with belt on elbows

Tips

✔ Press both outer elbows evenly down while lifting up the inner arms, the biceps and the deltoids. Keep this structure stable.

✔ Look at the elbows to check that they are equidistant from the center.

✔ Move the biceps up and forward (toward the triceps) and the shoulder blades in, toward the ribs. Attempt to increase the angle between the forearms and the upper arms toward 90°.

✔ Lift the biceps up and extend the triceps down to the front elbow; lift the inner arms up and cut the outer arms down to the outer elbows.

✔ When doing the pose without a belt on the elbows, make sure that they are not moving when you go up to the pose.

Sālamba Sirsāsana I

Variation 8
Lifting the shoulders: Using a support for the head

Effects
At first impression, it may appear that placing the head on a support compresses the neck; however, in many cases it enables one to lift the shoulders higher and thus to create length in the neck.

Props
blanket

In *Sirsāsana* one should lift the shoulder girdle as high as possible while keeping the crown of the head on the floor. For many people the shoulders can be lifted more easily when the head is slightly above the floor. This is especially true for those whose upper arms are long in proportion to the neck and head. Observe in photo ❶ how lifting the shoulders can lift the head off the floor.

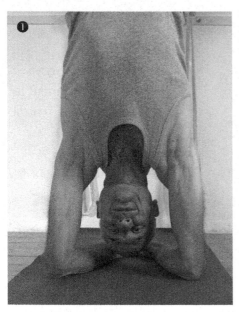

Lifting the head enables one to lift the shoulders higher

You can try it by doing the pose with the back to the wall about 10-15 cm (4-6 inches) away from it. Supporting the heels against the wall, lift up and check if the head lifts off the floor ❷.

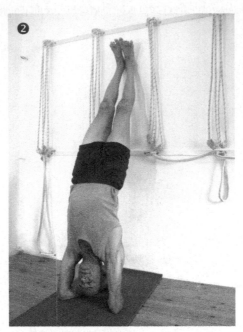

Lifting the head using the wall

However, having the crown of the head on the floor is an essential part of *Sirsāsana*. So, if your head lifts off the floor, you should fill that gap by supporting the head with a folded blanket. To measure the gap:

→ Kneel and place the head and the forearms on the floor as if going to *Sirsāsana* ❸.

❯ Push the floor and lift the shoulders as much as possible and allow the head to lift off the floor.

❯ Straighten the legs, step forward keeping the back concave.

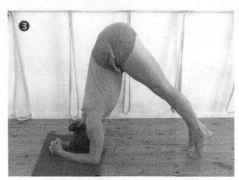

Measuring the gap between the head and the floor, when the shoulders are lifted

❯ Now, keeping the height of the shoulder girdle, release the neck to lower the head toward the floor.

❯ The moment your shoulder starts to drop, stop. Observe the gap between your head and the floor. This is the gap you have to fill with the blanket.

Using blanket support

The common way is to use a 3-folded blanket to support the head, so I show it first:

❯ Take a blanket folded as used for a *Sarvāngāsana* platform and 3-fold it.

❯ Place the 3-folded blanket on the mat and place the forearms on either side of the blanket.

❯ Interlock the fingers at the edge of the folded blanket, such that the forearms and outer edges of the hands are placed on the mat.

> Do not place the edge of the blanket on the palms, as this pushes the head forward while in the pose; leave a little gap between the blanket and the palms.

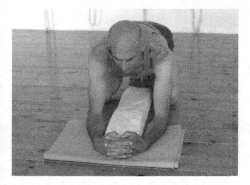

Adjusting a 3-folded blanket for head support

> Then go up to *Sirsāsana* maintaining the lift of the shoulders.

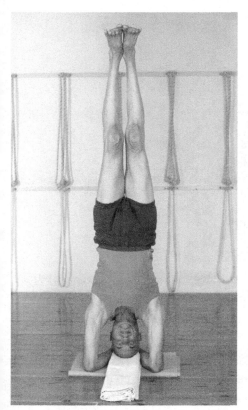

Sirsāsana on 3-folded blanket

Using a thinner blanket support

In some cases, a 3-folded blanket is too thick; the blanket can be folded into two or used without folding.

Using a 1-folded blanket:

→ Fold the edges of the blankets inward to allow the forearms to be on the floor.

> Place your head on the corner of the blanket, lift the shoulders and go up to *Sirsāsana*.

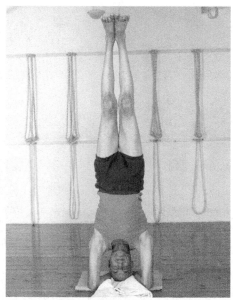

Sirsāsana on 1-folded blanket

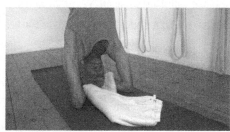

Sirsāsana on 2-folded blankets

You can also use a corner of a 2-folded blanket:

> Place the 2-folded blanket diagonally on the mat.

> Place the forearms on the mat, next to the corner of the blanket. Fold the blanket to allow the forearms to be on the mat.

> Press the forearms down, lift the shoulders and go up to the pose.

T i p s

✔ By all means avoid compression of the vulnerable cervical vertebrae – keep the shoulders lifted and the shoulder blades tucked in during the entire stay in the pose.

✔ If you are not sure yet about the height of the gap, start with a shallower support first.

✔ Press the forearms down to lift the upper arms. Connect the upper arms to the shoulder blades and the shoulder blades to the spine. At the same time stretch the legs up. Feel how these actions create an upward flow in the spine.

✔ Look forward at eye level with soft eyes and let the front brain recede toward the back brain.

Sālamba Sirsāsana I

Variation 9
Support the thoracic spine and
shoulder blades: Using blocks

Effects
The support for the upper back removes some load off the arms and neck; this makes it easier to open the chest, deepen the breath and stay longer in the pose. Feeling the proper position of the upper back, will help you to work toward it without support.

Props
several blocks
or chair,
wall, blanket
(optional)

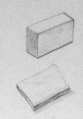

One of the challenges of *Sirsāsana* is to move the thoracic dorsal spine and the shoulder blades into the body. Failing to do so may create pressure on the vertebrae of the neck, which, over time, may lead to injury. When the arms are weak or injured, or the upper back is curved (excessive kyphosis), or the trapezius muscle is stiff - this action becomes difficult, and in some cases a support is needed. Even people who can do the pose independently will benefit from doing the pose with support from time to time.

The blocks can be arranged in several ways. Each person may need a slightly different arrangement, depending on his/her size and structure, the degree of movement in the shoulder girdle and the type of blocks used. I show here several possibilities. Please experiment to find out which one is most beneficial for you, or invent new modifications to suit your needs even better.

Supporting the thoracic dorsal spine

I. Using a block or two on top of a vertical block. people with long upper arms will need two blocks on top ❶, ❷ or ❸.

➡ Instead of interlocking the fingers, hold the bottom block firmly.

❯ Place the head about 5 cm (2 inches) away from the vertical block and go up to the pose.

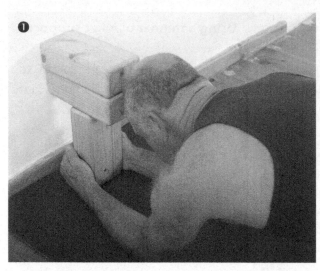

❶

Supporting the thoracic dorsal spine with two lowest-height blocks on top of a standing block

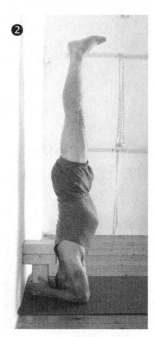

❷

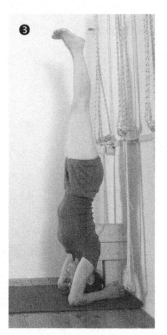

❸

Sirsāsana with blocks support – two lowest height blocks on top

Sirsāsana with blocks support – two second height blocks on top

T i p s

✓ Experiment to find the correct position of the head in relation to the vertical block. You should feel the blocks supporting the vertebrae in between the shoulder blades while the crown of the head rests on the floor. Excessive projection of the horizontal blocks makes it difficult to lift your legs into the pose.

II. Creating wider base by holding a lowest-height block

→ Place next to the wall a lowest-height block; place on it a highest-height block and on top a second-height block, whose edge against the wall ❹.

> Hold the lowest block and go up to *Sirsāsana*. Have the top block support the thoracic dorsal spine ❺.

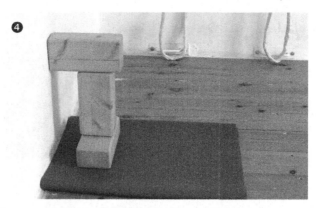

Lowest – highest – second-height blocks arrangement

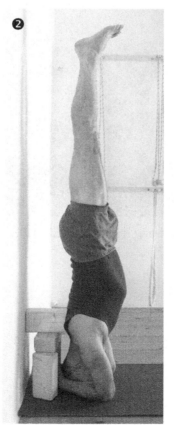

Sirsāsana with:
lowest – highest – second-height blocks arrangement

III. 'Bridge' structure for dorsal spine

→ Place the blocks in a 'bridge' structure ❶.

> Place the cup-shaped palms under that bridge.

> Go up to the pose. The fourth block on top supports the dorsal spine ❷.

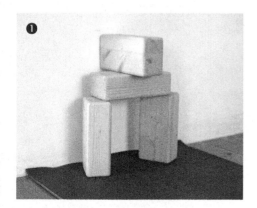

Using 4 blocks to create a 'bridge'

Sirsāsana with 'bridge' support for dorsal spine

Note:

In some cases, the support for the upper back tends to lift the head off the floor. In this case, support the head with a folded blanket as shown in Variation 8 on page 23.

Sālamba Sirsāsana I

Variation 9 (Cont'd)
Support the thoracic spine and shoulder blades: Using blocks

Supporting the shoulder blades

<u>I. 'Bridge' structure</u>

Here you need five blocks.

→ Use three blocks to make a bridge, and place two second-height blocks on top ❶.

> The distance between the two top blocks should match the distance between your shoulder blades.

Go up to the pose where the two top blocks support the shoulder blades ❷.

<u>II. T-shape</u>

Here you need 4 blocks.

→ Use two blocks in a T-shape and place two blocks on top of the T ❸.

> The distance between the two top blocks should match the distance between your shoulder blades.

> Instead of interlocking the fingers hold the bottom (vertical) block ❹.

Note: Place the two top blocks simultaneously; otherwise the structure will lose its balance and collapse.

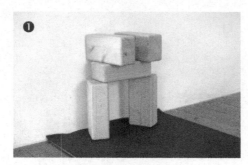
Forming a 'bridge' from 5 blocks

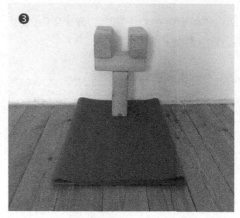
Two blocks on a T-shape

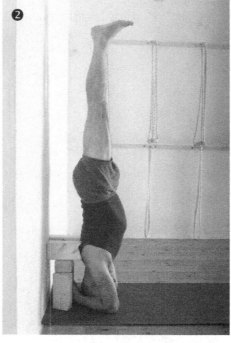
Sirsāsana with 'bridge' support for shoulder blades

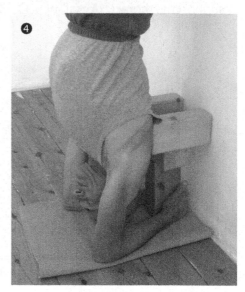
Sirsāsana supporting the shoulder blades with 4 blocks

Applicability

All the Sirsāsana variations; especially Pārśva Sirsāsana and Eka Pāda Sirsāsana.

Sālamba Sirsāsana I

Variation 10
Supporting the shoulder blades: Using a chair

Effects

The chair stabilizes the shoulder blades and helps to maintain their balance and alignment. In the inverted chair option, it also gives a framework for the elbows. Pressing the elbows against the backrest activates the arms.

Props

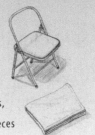

chair,

<u>optional:</u>

wall, blankets, sticky mat pieces

Here are two ways of using the chair, try both to see which is more helpful for the shape of your body.

I. Inverted chair

→ Invert the chair and place it next to the wall.

❯ If you find that the support of the seat is lower than your shoulder blades, then lift the chair on blocks ❶ (or foam blocks).

> **Note:** Placing the legs of the chair against the wall prevents it from slipping off the blocks.

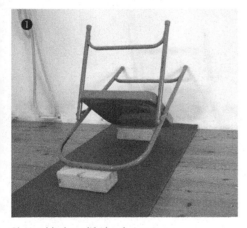

Placing blocks to lift the chair

❯ Place the elbows against the framework of the backrest and go up to the pose, using the seat to support the shoulder blades ❷.

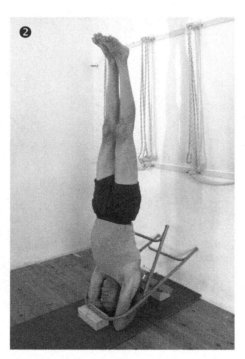

Sirsāsana with inverted chair

❯ If the shoulder blades are not well supported by the seat, then probably the distance is too large – in this case pad the seat with some folded blankets ❸.

❯ If the width of the backrest is bigger than the width of your shoulders, pad the backrest with folded sticky mats (or pieces) ❹.

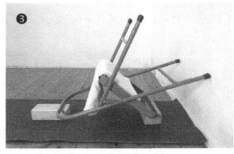

Padding the seat of the chair

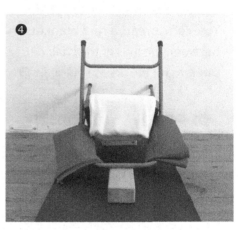

Padding the seat and the backrest

Tips

✔ Work the elbows against the backrest of the chair to activate the upper arms.

✔ Lift the inner sides of the upper arms and widen the collar bones.

✔ The seat of the chair should support the shoulder blades and move them in (forward).

Variation 10 (Cont'd)
Supporting the shoulder blades:
Using a chair

II. Using the edge of the seat

⟶ Place the chair against the wall and use the front edge of the seat as a support for the shoulder blades.

❯ For most people, the seat is higher than the shoulder girdle; in this case do the pose on an elevated platform. You can spread a few blankets in between the legs of the chair or use three foam blocks as shown in ❺.

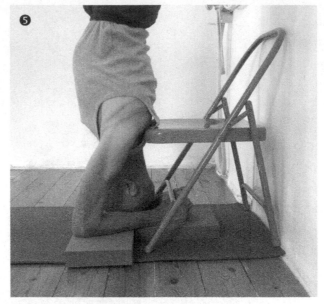

❺

Support the shoulders by the seat of the chair

T i p s

✔ Learn to press the outer corner of the wrists firmly to the floor.

✔ If the chair tends to fold, then use a belt to tie it as shown on page XVI.

Applicability

Most Sirsāsana variations; especially Pārśva Sirsāsana, Eka Pāda Sirsāsana and Pārśvaika Pāda Sirsāsana.

Sālamba Sirsāsana I

Variation 11
Supporting the shoulder blades: Using the bottom rope

Effects

The rope helps to keep the shoulder blades lifted and stable.

Props

bottom wall hook, rope

→ Attach a long rope to a bottom (floor-level) hook.

> **Note:** If the rope is not long enough, connect a second rope to it.

❯ Stand above the loop of the rope and bend forward **❶**.

❯ Insert the head and arms into the loop and place the rope on the shoulder blades **❷**.

❯ Keeping the rope against the upper back, place the forearms on the mat and interlock the fingers. Move away from the wall until the rope is well stretched **❸**.

❯ Now lift one leg at a time to *Sirsāsana* **❹**.

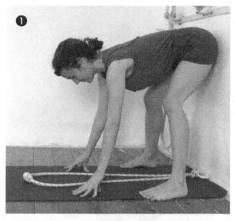

Entering into the loop attached to a bottom hook – stage 1

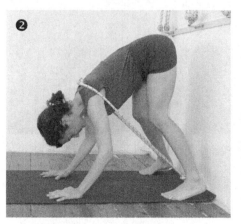

Entering into the loop attached to a bottom hook – stage 2

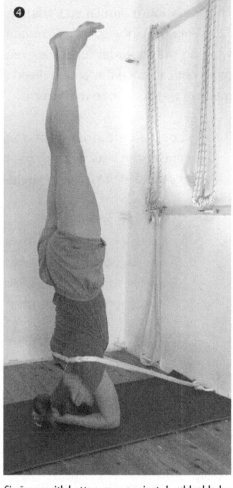

Sirsāsana with bottom rope against shoulder blades

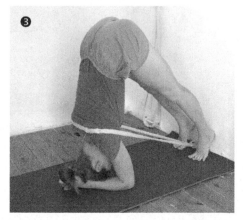

Entering into the loop attached to a bottom hook – stage 3

Applicability:

All the Sirsāsana variations. Especially Pārśva Sirsāsana and Eka Pāda Parivṛtta Sirsāsana (see the section on "Sirsāsana Cycle"). If your back is supple you can also arch back to Dwi Pāda Viparīta Dandāsana using the support of the rope.

Sālamba Sirsāsana I

Variation 12
Sensing the shoulder blades:
Belt around chest

Effects

The touch of the belt brings awareness to the top chest and shoulder blades. It helps to move the shoulder blades in, and to sense their symmetry.

Props

belt

This Variation is similar to Variation 12 in Volume 1; however, in *Sirsāsana* working the shoulder blades is even more critical, since this action diverts much of the body load to the arms.

→ Loop a belt around the top chest and fasten it such that the belt touches the skin but is not too tight.

> ### *T i p s*
> ✔ If a helper is available she or he can move your shoulder blades down and in before tightening the belt. This improves the shoulder blades action.

❯ Go up to *Sirsāsana*.

> ### *T i p s*
> ✔ Move both shoulder blades away from the belt and the manubrium bone (top sternum) toward the belt.
>
> ✔ Lift the top chest as if trying to lift the belt.

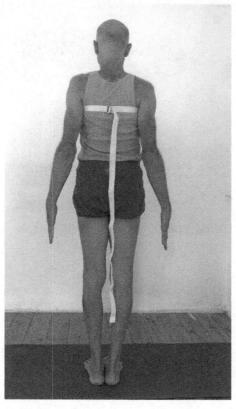

Placing a belt on the chest

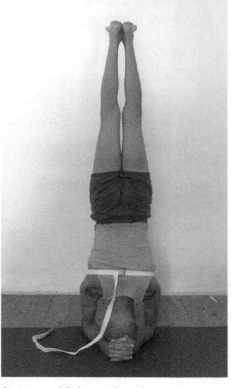

Sirsāsana with belt around top chest

Correct Positioning of the Head

Sālamba Sirsāsana I

Variation 13
Sensing the head orientation:
A block against the back of the head

Effects

The block helps to stabilize the head and to sense its orientation. A correct vertical alignment of the head ensures an even circulation to the front and the rear parts of the brain. This brings about a special sensation of quietude and coolness. The eyes recede and the pose becomes more meditative.

This Variation is also helpful for people who, for some reason, cannot interlock the fingers and support the head with the palms.

Props

block

Beginners tend to balance their *Sirsāsana* on a region between the crown of the head and the forehead. However, as explained above, the full benefit of the pose is achieved when the skull is exactly vertical, such that an imaginary plumb line can be drawn from the crown of the head through the perineum to the meeting point of the two ankles.

Look at somebody doing *Sirsāsana* from the side. Observe the longitudinal line of the ear: if it is vertical then the head is positioned properly. When doing the pose alone, you may not know exactly how the head is positioned. In order to develop that sensitivity, you can use a block.

→ Instead of interlocking the fingers, hold a block and place it against the occiput (the back of the skull).

❯ Go up to *Sirsāsana* and keep pulling the block with the fingers to hold it firmly against the occiput.

Try to roll the head slightly backward and balance on the rear part of the crown of the head.

Observe the effect on the brain and the mind when you find the correct spot.

> **Tips**
> ✔ If the block is not supporting the middle of the back of the skull, lift it slightly with your fingers (as shown in photo).

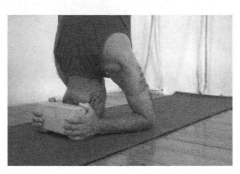

Sirsāsana with block against the back of the head

> ⚠ **CAUTIONS**
> 1. Do not move the head when in the pose as this may injure the neck. In order to correct the alignment of the head, go down, place the head properly, and go up again.
>
> 2. Do not attempt to straighten the neck completely. The natural curvature (lordosis) of the neck should be maintained.

> **Tips**
> ✔ Allow the eyeballs to soften and recede into their sockets. Look forward, parallel to the floor, with a soft, non-focused gaze.
>
> ✔ See that the crown (top) of the brain is not pushed into the crown (top) of the skull, but imagine it is being lifted toward the center of the chest. The brain cells should not feel compressed or heated.
>
> ✔ Guruji Iyengar said that the brain should feel cool in *Sirsāsana* – do you feel that?

Sālamba Sirsāsana I

Variation 14
Sensing the head orientation:
A belt under top of head

Some people tend to tilt or turn the head to one side. The belt helps to sense
and correct this.

belt

→ Stretch a belt along the center of the mat.

❯ Place the top of the head on the edge of the belt and go up to the pose.

❯ Look forward and make sure your eyes are following the line of the belt.

❯ Close one eye at a time and check if the images you get from each eye are symmetrical.

Tips
✔ Feel the belt under your head and make sure it is exactly under the center of the top of the head.

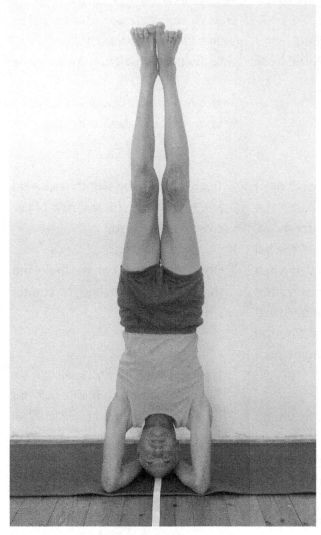

Sirsāsana with a belt under the top of the head

Help in Lifting the Shoulders

Lifting the shoulders is a crucial action in *Sirsāsana*. If you do not maintain the shoulder girdle lifted at all times when staying in the pose, you risk your cervical vertebrae and you also create compression in the eyes and ears. This will reduce the great benefit that *Sirsāsana* has on these sense organs. The brain cells also should not feel compressed; otherwise instead of joy you will experience stress. The Variations in this section use props to lift the shoulders. Once you experience that, you will be able to work better in order to create this effect without props.

Sālamba Sirsāsana I

Variation 15
Lifting the shoulders:
Helpers pulling ropes

Effects
The pull of the ropes lifts the shoulders; this combined with the grounding of the forearms extends the neck and makes the pose feel light.

Props
two ropes, two helpers, wall (optional)

In this Variation, each helper lifts one shoulder of the practitioner while pressing the corresponding forearm down. The helpers should synchronize their actions as mirror images of each other.

> **Note:** Do the pose with the back to the wall, since the pull of the helpers may tilt you out of balance.

Instructions for the helpers:

→ Once the practitioner is in *Sirsāsana* with the back to the wall, stand to his/her side. Insert the rope between the practitioner's neck and shoulder.

> Place the arch of your foot on the practitioner's forearm and gently ground it to the floor while pulling the rope diagonally up and towards you.

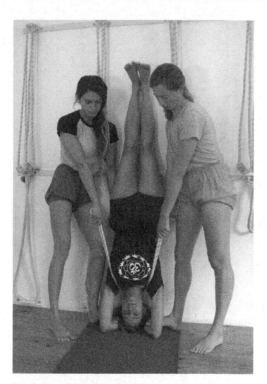

Two helpers lifting the shoulders

T i p s (for the helpers):

✔ Be extra careful not to exert too much pressure on the forearm of the practitioner.

✔ Synchronize your pull with that of the other helper (ask the practitioner if the pull feels equal on both sides).

Applicability:
The same pull is a very helpful in Pīncha Mayurāsana and Adho Mukha Vṛkṣāsana.

Sālamba Sirsāsana I

Variation 16
Lifting the shoulders:
Helper uses his/her shin bones

Effects

The lift of the shoulders and the trapezius allows extending and releasing the neck. This clarifies the action of lifting and broadening the shoulders in Sirsāsana.

Props

one helper

Here the helper uses his shin bones as rods for lifting the shoulders of the practitioner (see Variation 31 on page 54 for using rods to support the trapezius). Instructions for the helper:

→ After the practitioner has placed her/his forearms and head on the floor, sit behind her/him and carefully insert your feet and shins in the gaps between the practitioner's forearms and upper arms.

❯ Place your shins in the spaces between the neck and the shoulders of the practitioner and gently move your shins to lift his/her shoulders ❶.

❯ When the practitioner goes up to *Sirsāsana* support his/her back and keep lifting his/her shoulders, without pushing him/her forward ❷.

> **Note:** If the practitioner is not stable, then sit with your back against the wall. This allows the practitioner to lean his/her heels on the wall, in case he/she loses balance ❸.

❯ After a while, you can slowly withdraw your legs and allow the practitioner to stay in the pose independently, attempting to maintain the same lift of the trapezius and shoulders.

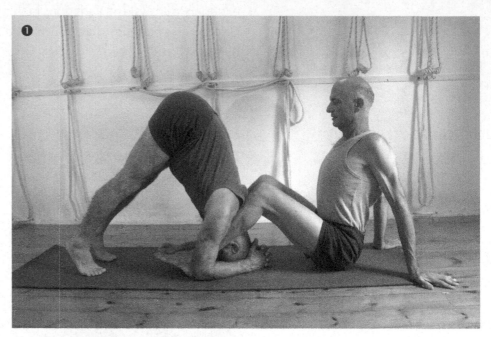

A helper lifts the shoulders with his shins – stage 1

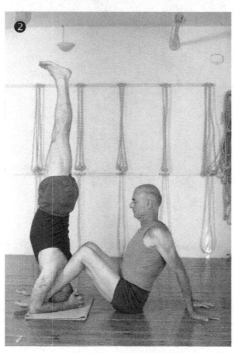

A helper lifts the shoulders with his shins – final stage

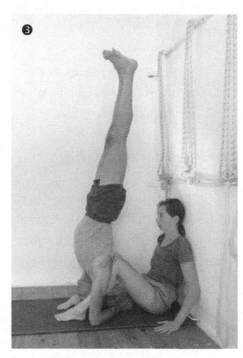

A helper lifts the shoulders with his shins – next to the wall

Sālamba Sirsāsana I

Variation 17
Lifting the shoulders:
Belt from heels to shoulder girdle

Effects
The rope that embraces the shoulder girdle is pulled by the heels; this helps to lift the shoulders. This is similar to the shoulder traction shown in Variation 11 of Tadāsana in Volume I (page 15), but in Sirsāsana these effects are more critical and more difficult to achieve. Pulling the shoulders up using the strength of the legs relieves compression of the cervical region and helps to learn this action.

Props
rope, long belt

→ Wrap a rope around the shoulder girdle as shown in Variation 11 of *Tadāsana* (see ❶ here). Insert a long belt in the loop of the rope (adjust the length of the belt as explained for *Tadāsana*).

❯ Kneel and get ready for *Sirsāsana*. Hook one heel in the belt and stretch it.

❯ Go up to *Sirsāsana* while you keep stretching the belt with one heel ❷. Once you are in the pose ❸, insert the other heel into the loop of the belt.

❶
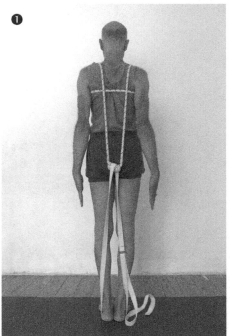
Shoulder traction in *Tadāsana*

❷
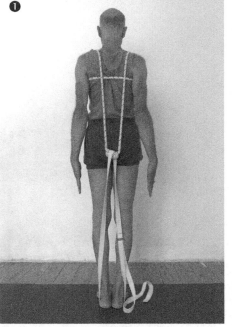
Coming up - hooking one heel

❸
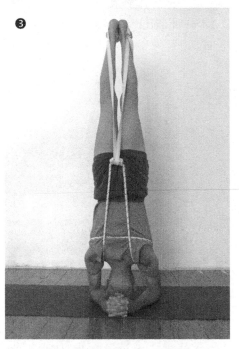
Stretch the legs up to lift the trapezius muscles

❹
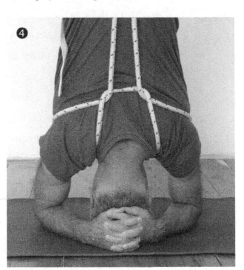
Shoulder traction in *Sirsāsana*

Activating the Legs

Sālamba Sirsāsana I

Variation 18
Activating the legs:
Block between thighs

Effects

The block activates the legs and helps to turn the thighs inward. It also creates width in the pelvis and the lower abdomen and helps to move the lumbar spine backward.

Props

block, belt
(optional)

→ Hold a block between the thighs and go up to *Sirsāsana*.

❯ Press the block firmly, and attempt to lift it.

❯ Roll the thighs from outside in, as if to move the block backward.

❯ Move the tailbone in and up (toward the block). Lift the buttock bones up toward the heels.

Notes:

1. If you are not stable in the pose, use a soft block (rubber or cork rather than wood) to soften the impact in case it falls.

2. If you cannot go up with a block between the thighs, ask someone to place the block for you once you are in the pose.

Tips

✔ Move the back groins outward and observe how the skin of the buttocks broadens as if to embrace the pelvis.

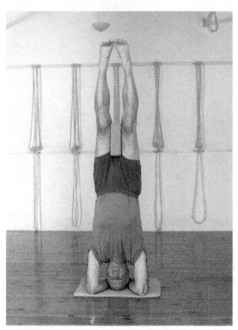

Sirsāsana with block between the thighs

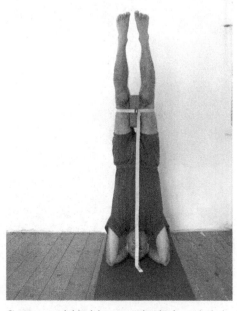

Sirsāsana with block between the thighs and a belt

Using a belt to encircle the thighs

Effects: Here the widening of the pelvic girdle is combined with the compactness gained from the belt, and the effort to hold the pose is reduced. Women in advanced pregnancy should do Sirsāsana in this way.

→ Hold the block between the thighs and tighten a belt around the thighs.

Tips

✔ Place the buckle in the middle, between the thighs and use the dropped tail of the belt as a plumb line to gauge your alignment and stability. The belt should extend down in line with the nose and the center of the forehead. Watch the movements of the belt to learn about the movements of your legs. Try to stabilize the pose until the belt comes to stillness.

Sālamba Sirsāsana I

Variation 19
Activating the legs: Bracing the legs

Effects

The belts sharpen the awareness at the feet and thus help to broaden and lift them. Sense the touch of the buckle on the feet and lift it up!

Props

belts, rolled mat (optional)

Belts can be used to brace the legs at various positions – each producing a different effect. I show here several options for your experimentation. Enjoy!

> **Note:** In these Variations you will not be able to go up to the pose one leg after the other, but you can go up with bent knees.

I. Belt around ankles and lower legs

Effects: The belts on the ankles and lower legs help to roll the tarsal and metatarsals bones inward and to stabilize the legs, thus making the entire pose more stable.

II. Belt around the big toes

Effects: Using a belt to join the big toes is especially useful for people who cannot spread the toes and join the big toes. Some people have a protuberance in the joints of the big toes (hallux valgus) and they cannot move the big toe away from the second toe. Tying the big toes gives them a sense of alignment and stability in the pose.

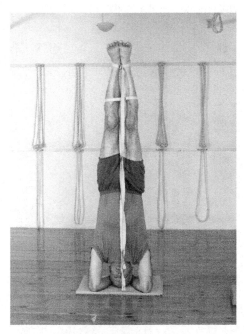

Sirsāsana - belts around ankles and shins

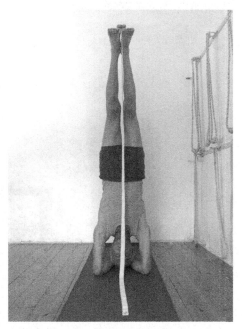

Sirsāsana - belt around big toes

Tips

✔ Extend from the inner arches of the feet both forward (toward the big toes) and backward (toward the inner heels).

Variation 19 (Cont'd)
Activating the legs: Bracing the legs

III. Belt forming a 'sandal'

Effects: *The crossing of the belts braces the two feet to each other; this stabilizes the legs and induces serenity. It also joins the big toes together, as in the previous option.*

➡️ Cross an open belt around the big toes ❶.

❯ Then cross the two edges over and then under the feet ❷.

❯ And finally cross behind the lower legs and tighten the belt ❸.

❯ Go up to *Sirsāsana* with the crossed belt ❹.

T i p s

✔ Activate the legs by widening the feet against the resistance of the belt.

✔ Lift the inner edges of the feet and broaden the toes from inside out as if to stretch the belt.

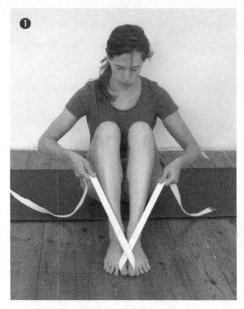

Wrapping the belt as a 'sandal' – stage 1

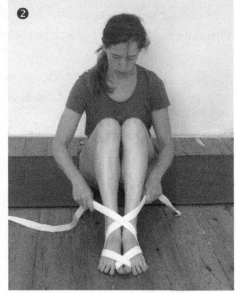

Wrapping the belt as a 'sandal' – stage 2

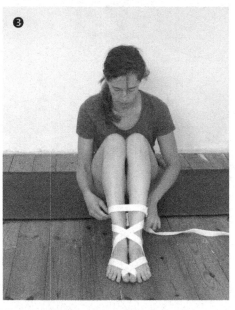

Wrapping the belt as a 'sandal' – stage 3

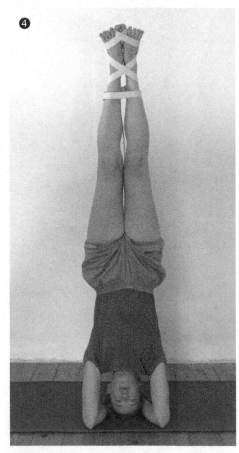

Sirsāsana - belt crossed from toes to ankles (as a sandal)

IV. Six belts and a rolled mat

Effects: *This is an excellent work for people who suffer from minor deformities in the legs (like 'O' or 'X' shaped legs). It relieves knee pain. Persistent practice will improve the alignment of the long bones of the legs and of the knees.*

This is similar to Variation 7 of *Dandāsana* (see Volume 2 p. 11).

→ Sit in *Dandāsana*. Loop 6 belts around the legs as explained in Volume 2.

❯ Roll a mat and insert it in between the legs, then tighten the belts.

❯ Go up to *Sirsāsana*.

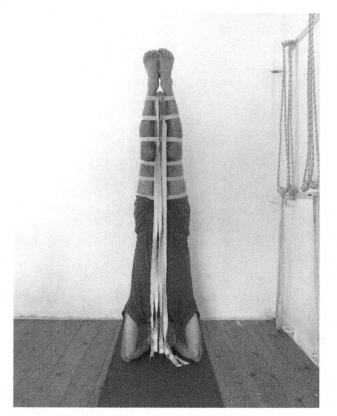

Sirsāsana - rolled mat and 6 belts

Applicability:
The same arrangement can be used in other poses with straight and joined legs, such as Sālamba Sarvāngāsana, Ūrdhva Prasārita Pādāsana and Dandāsana.

Sālamba Sirsāsana I

Variation 20
Lifting the buttocks:
Belts from pelvis to heels

Effects

The belts around the pelvis create compactness in the hips and alertness in the pelvis and legs. Pulling the belts with the heels lifts the buttocks and activates the legs. This helps to learn this action. It is a boon for people who suffer from lower back pain in Sirsāsana.

Props

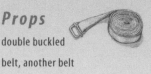

double buckled belt, another belt

Note: a double buckled belt has a second buckle on its end which is used to connect to a regular (single buckled) belt.

Lifting the buttocks upward is an important action of *Sirsāsana*. However, since these regions of the body are at the back, the awareness there is often dull and the buttocks tend to stick out and fall toward the lumbar. This may create pressure on the lower back.

➡️ Tighten the double buckled belt around the pelvis such that its loose end points inwards.

❯ Tighten another (regular) belt opposite to it. Adjust the belts such that the buckles are on either sides of the sacrum.

❯ Reach the arms behind the back and tighten the two belts evenly ❶.

❯ Now connect the loose end of the regular belt to the second buckle of the double buckle belt and adjust the length of the loop such that it hangs near the floor ❷.

Note: You can use two regular belts by tying their loose ends with a knot. But this makes it much harder to adjust the length of the loop.

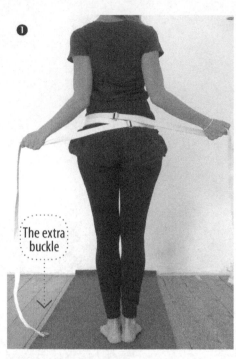

The extra buckle

Tightening the belts in opposite directions

❯ Stand in *Tadāsana*, bend the knees and tighten the loop. When you straighten the legs, the belts should be well stretched and you should feel the pull on the buttocks.

❯ After adjusting the loop, go up to *Sirsāsana*, using one heel to stretch the belts, as explained in Variation 17 above.

❯ In *Sirsāsana* stretch the legs up to lift the buttocks toward the heels ❸. Soften the abdominal organs and allow them to recede toward the diaphragm.

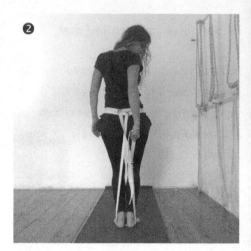

Adjusting the belt

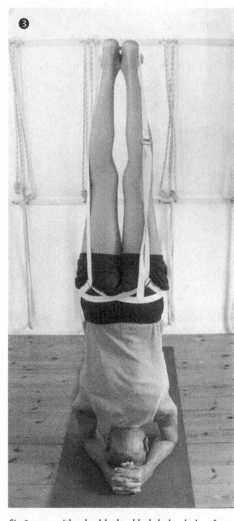

Sirsāsana with double-buckled belt; belts from pelvis to heels

Sālamba Sirsāsana I

Variation 21
Activating and stabilizing the legs: A pen between the toes and a pendulum

Effects
The word 'sthira' in yoga sutra 2.46 (sthira sukham āsanam), means stability, firmness, stillness or steadiness. The more stability you experience in an āsana, the greater are its benefits. Two ways are given to check and improve the stability of Sirsāsana: holding a pen between the big toes and hanging a small weight on the feet. Both direct awareness to the legs, feet and toes. The pen between the toes also teaches how to spread the toes.

Props
pen,

optional: helper and a piece of paper.

Or: a small weight and a long belt

Using a pen:

Hold a pen in between the big toes and go up to *Sirsāsana* ❶. To do so, you must keep the legs joined, but you may bend them to come up.

T i p s
✔ Learn to create space between the big toe and the second toe.

✔ Imagine there is a piece of paper right above your feet (or ask a friend to hold an actual piece of paper for you ❷). Your mission is to draw a single dot. If the legs sway they will leave a scribble on the page.

✔ Learn to stabilize the legs (*sthira*). Reduce to a minimum their movements; the pose will then become much quieter.

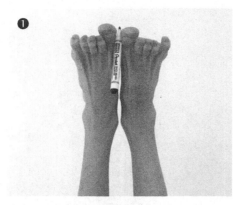
❶

Sirsāsana - holding a pen between the big toes

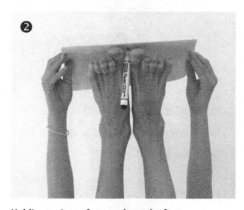
❷

Holding a piece of paper above the feet

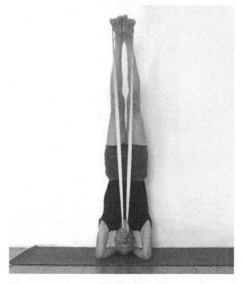

Sirsāsana with a small weight used as a pendulum

Using a weight as a pendulum:

A small metal weight hung on the feet acts as a pendulum to reflect the movements of the legs.

Connect a weight of 2-3 kg (4-6 lbs.) to the belt and adjust the length of the belt such that when you are in the pose, the weight will be hung in front of your face.

❯ Insert one foot in the loop of the belt and come up to *Sirsāsana*. Then insert the other foot in the loop.

> *Note:* Coming up to *Sirsāsana* this way is a bit of a challenge; if a helper is available ask her/him to hang the weight on you once you are in the pose.

❯ Now stabilize the legs until the weight becomes still. Keep observing the weight and monitor its movements; learn to be still and quiet in the pose.

Sālamba Sīrsāsana I

Variation 22
Activating the legs:
Helper pulls a rope placed in between the inner thighs

Effects

Pulling the rope sensitizes the inner thighs and helps to lengthen and lift the inner legs. The legs become more active when squeezing against the rope. The upward pull makes the pose light and demonstrates the role of the legs in Sīrsāsana.

Props

rope or belt,
chair, helper

Instructions for the helper:

⟶ Once the practitioner is up in *Sirsāsana*, place a chair behind her/him, and stand on it holding the rope.

❯ Ask the practitioner to slightly spread her/his legs and hang the rope in between her/his legs, such that the knot is placed between the practitioner's upper thighs.

❯ Now ask the practitioner to join the legs and hold the rope in between the legs. Optionally you can tighten a belt around the practitioner's thighs to keep them joined tightly ❶.

❯ Gently pull the rope up. The practitioner should tighten her/his legs attempting to prevent the rope from sliding upward.

> *Note:* If there is a large gap between the practitioner's thighs, then insert the rope under the belt and pull its two edges upward, evenly ❷.

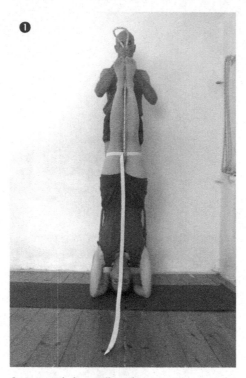

❶

Sirsāsana - helper pulling the rope up against the resistance of the practitioners legs

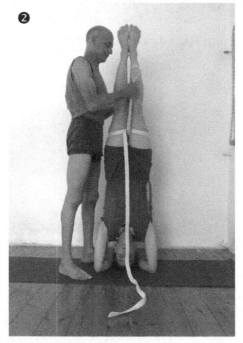

❷

Another way of lifting the inner legs

Tips

✔ Stretch the legs to lift the bones of the pelvis, while completely releasing the abdominal organs which are dropped back (toward the lumbar) and down (toward the diaphragm).

✔ Feel how the diaphragmatic breath massages the abdominal organs.

Sālamba Sirsāsana I

Variation 23
Activating the legs:
Helpers pull the groins down

Often it is easier to activate muscles against a resistance which clarifies the direction in which the muscles should work. Once this is learnt, the muscles can be activated in the same way even without the resistance. In Sirsāsana one needs to lift the pelvis by stretching the legs upward. It is not always clear which muscles should work and how; after all, we are used to activating the legs against the resistance of the floor (or the gravity of the earth) and not to stretch them upward into the air. In this Variation the legs and the buttocks are stretching upward, against the downward vertical pull of the groins.

Props

two ropes (or belts), two helpers

This and the following Variations are examples of prop usages that make the pose more difficult, rather than providing some support or relief. But, by creating resistance, the props teach the body to act in the desired direction (as I already mentioned, it is easier to push against a resistance than to push 'the air').

Instruction for the helpers:

→ Once the practitioner is in *Sirsāsana*, ask her/him to spread the legs slightly.

› Place a rope on each groin and gently pull the two ends of the rope vertically down.

› The practitioner then joins the legs and extends them up.

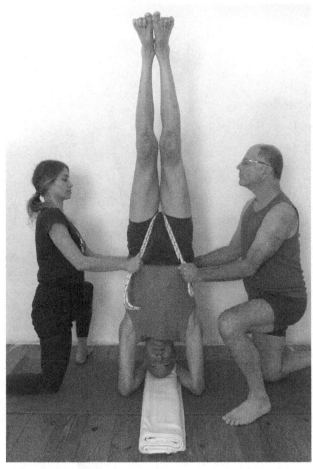

Sirsāsana - two helpers pull the groins down

Tips

✓ Helpers: Ask the practitioner if the intensity of the pull is appropriate and if it is even on both sides. Adjust accordingly.

✓ Practitioner: Lift the inner legs up from the groins, and at the same time keep the abdominal organs soft; allow these organs to recede back toward the spine.

Sālamba Sirsāsana I

Variation 24
Activating the legs:
Hanging weight on the heels

Effects

The weight teaches how to align the legs and the spine vertically (if the legs are tilted it becomes very difficult to carry the weight). The weight also strengthens the bones of the legs, which extend against the resistance.

Props

weight of 5 - 10 kg
(10 - 20 lbs.), helper

 CAUTIONS
Start with 5 kg (10 lbs.), and only if you feel safe try to increase the weight.

This is an advanced variation that can be done only if:

- You are stable and secure in *Sirsāsana*, and able to lift the shoulders well and stay in the pose for at least 10 minutes

- A trained helper is available to place the weight on your heels while you are in the pose.

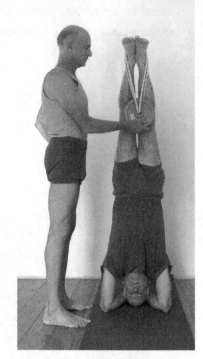

Sirsāsana - placing weight on the heels

Instructions for the helper:

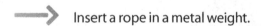 Insert a rope in a metal weight.

> *Note:* You can use a sand bag instead of a metal weight; this is safer in the beginning.

> Once the practitioner is in the pose, carefully place the rope on her/his heels while holding the weight in your other hand.

> Slowly lower the weight until it is hanging on the heels of the practitioner.

> Stand near the practitioner and be ready to remove the weight whenever necessary.

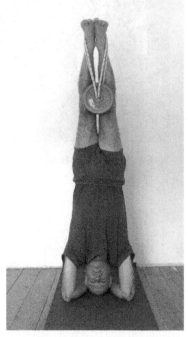

Sirsāsana - with weight hanging from the heels

Tips

✔ Extend and lift the bones of the legs against the resistance. Extend the bones as if to touch the inner heels – keep this contact as long as you are in the pose.

Sirsāsana Cycle

In *Light on Yoga* Guruji Iyengar wrote on the *Sirsāsana* Cycle:

"In Sirsasana there is a variety of movements which can be practised at one stretch after staying in Salamba Sirsasana for not less than 5 minutes…"

The variations done in the cycle enhance the effects of the *āsana*.

Sālamba Sirsāsana I

Variation 25
Checking the alignment in *Pārśva Sirsāsana* and *Eka Pāda Sirsāsana*: Back to the wall

Effects
The wall teaches the vertical alignment of the body in Sirsāsana (provided that the gap between the head and the wall is minimal). This is good way to gauge the alignment in Sirsāsana variations like: Eka Pāda Sirsāsana (LOY Pl. 208), Parśvaika Pāda Sirsāsana (LOY Pl. 210 - not shown here) and Pārśva Sirsāsana (LOY Pl. 202).

Props
wall

In the variations of *Sirsāsana I*, it is challenging to keep correct alignment and extension.

→ Stand in *Sirsāsana I* with your back against the wall.

Proceed to *Pārśva Sirsāsana*:

> Turn the pelvis and the legs to the right. At the same time cut the outer right armpit forward (away from the wall) and move the right collar bone toward the left collar bone.

> Do not allow the face and chest to turn to the right.

> Keep lifting the left leg from its root and turn it from outside in.

> Turn the pelvis and legs more until the outer right foot touches the wall.

> Keep the legs vertical and extend them up.

> Come back to *Sirsāsana I* and do the pose to the left.

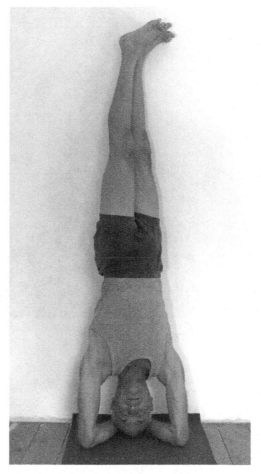

Pārśva Sirsāsana – back to the wall

Tips
✔ When doing the pose to the right: sharpen the forward gaze of the right eye; this prevents the head from turning to the right.

Sālamba Sirsāsana I

Variation 25 (Cont'd)
Checking the alignment in *Pārśva Sirsāsana* and *Eka Pāda Sirsāsana*: Back to the wall

Proceed to *Eka Pāda Sirsāsana*:

→ Lean your buttocks and heels against the wall.

❭ Keeping the right buttock in contact with the wall, lower the right leg until it is parallel to the floor.

❭ Stretch the leg forward and move the heel away from the wall; at the same time keep the contact of the right femur bone with the pelvis.

❭ Extend the inner right leg from the groin to the inner heel and open the foot.

❭ At the same time, move the outer right thigh back to the wall. The right hip and right outer ankle should be in line (the right foot should not move toward the center of the body).

❭ Keep the left heel on the wall. Keep extending that leg up and do not allow it to turn outward.

❭ Keeping these actions move the buttocks slightly away from the wall. Keep both buttocks at the same height and equidistant from the wall.

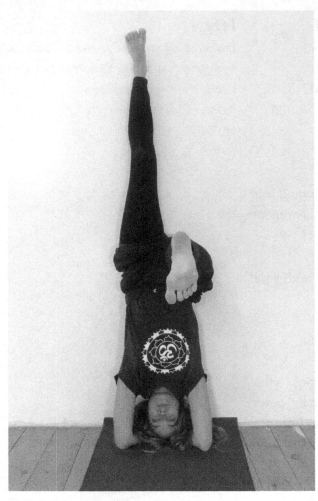

Eka Pāda Sirsāsana - back to the wall

Tips

✓ To verify the correct position of the pelvis, move it toward the wall and sense if both buttocks touch the wall concurrently and leveled.

Sālamba Sirsāsana I

Variation 26
Eka Pāda Sirsāsana and *Parśvaika Pāda Sirsāsana*: Lowered foot on chair

Effects

The chairs provides support for the lowered leg and hence enable one to stay longer in the pose and to improve the alignment of the pelvis region.

Props

2 -3 chairs

→ Place one chair in front (for *Eka Pāda Sirsāsana*), and the two other chairs on the left and right (for *Parśvaika Pāda Sirsāsana*).

Notes:

1. You can use chairs of any kind, but they should have the same height.

2. If you do not have three chairs, do first *Eka Pāda* with one chair, then go down and arrange two chairs for *Parśvaika Pāda* (or ask someone to do that for you).

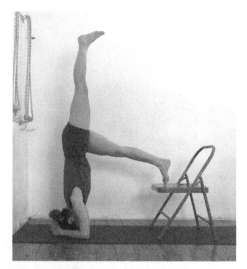

Eka Pāda Sirsāsana - lowered foot on chair

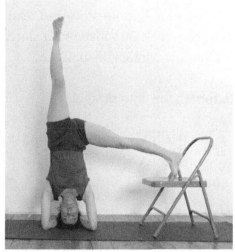

Parśvaika Pāda Sirsāsana - lowered foot on chair

Proceed to *Eka Pāda Sirsāsana*:

> From *Sirsāsana* lower the right leg to place the tips of the toes on the chair.

> Press the toes against the seat and lift the front thigh.

> Keep the left leg well stretched vertically up and do not allow it to turn outward.

> Do not drop the right side of the pelvis or allow it to move forward – the pelvis should remain aligned.

> Then lift the right leg and repeat on the left.

Proceed to *Parśvaika Pāda Sirsāsana*:

> Turn the right leg out and align its heel with the center of the arch of the left foot.

> Lower the right leg laterally to place the tips of the toes on the seat of the chair.

> Press the toes against the chair and lift the front thigh.

> Tuck the right buttock in and keep the pelvis aligned.

Tips

✔ When moving the leg down, stretch the leg to the heel, and at the same time keep the foot close to the body. The femur bone should be moving toward the hip socket.

✔ Keep both buttock bones in line and leveled.

Variation 27
Pārśva Sirsāsana using a chair

Effects

The edge of the seat gives a sharp sensation in the shoulder blades region. When turning sideways, avoid the tendency of the opposite shoulder blade to move away from the chair.

Props

chair, wall

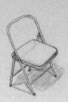

This Variation is more advanced than using the wall (as in Variation 25), since one has to maintain the balance.

To turn to the right side:

→ Place a chair with its back against the wall (see Variation 10 on page 28).

❯ If the seat of the chair is higher than your shoulder blades, then do the pose on a raised platform (made of several foam blocks or folded blankets).

❯ Place the cup-shaped palms under the chair.

❯ Go up to *Sirsāsana*.

> **Note:** Verify that the edge of the seat supports the shoulder blades. If necessary, go down to adjust the position of the forearms to achieve this.

❯ Now turn the pelvis and the legs to the right.

❯ Tuck the right shoulder blade in (away from the chair) and turn the upper chest from right to left. Maintain the back side of the left shoulder in contact with the chair.

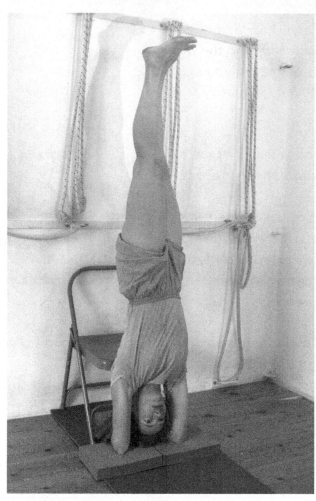

Pārśva Sirsāsana – shoulder blades against a chair

Sālamba Sirsāsana I

Variation 28
Learning Ūrdhva Padmāsana: Using the wall

Effects

Crossing the legs to Padmāsana when in Sirsāsana (Ūrdhva Padmāsana in Sirsāsana – LOY Pl. 211) is challenging for many people, since the hands cannot be used to help in crossing the legs. Using the floor and/or a wall corner enables you to use the hands for this action.

Props
wall

> ⚠️ **CAUTIONS**
>
> As in all *Padmāsana* variations exercise special care not to injure the knees. If you already have an injured knee, avoid this variation and consult an experienced Iyengar Yoga teacher.

Here are two options:

I. Lowering one leg to the floor

→ Do *Sirsāsana*, optionally with your back against the wall.

> Bend the right leg into *Ardha* (half) *Padmāsana* .

> Then, keeping the right foot on the left groin, lower the left leg down to the floor and use your left hand to move the right foot to its position ❷.

> Now lift the right knee as much as possible to create space for the left foot ❸.

> *Note:* Repeat this stage several times, bending one leg, lowering the other one and moving the bent knee back. This is critical for *Padmāsana* – the leg you bend first must create space for the folding of the second leg. Do not continue to full *Padmāsana* before this is achieved.

> Now bend the left leg and place the foot on the top of the right thigh ❹.

> Lift the legs up, move the mid-buttocks in and the knees back (toward the wall). Lift the knees and draw them closer to each other ❺.

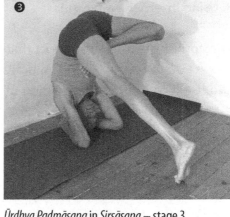

Ūrdhva Padmāsana in Sirsāsana – stage 3

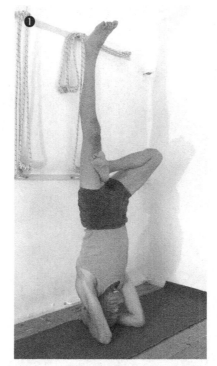

Ūrdhva Padmāsana in Sirsāsana – stage 1

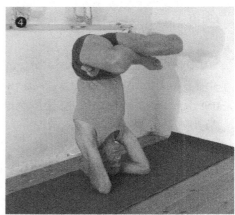

Ūrdhva Padmāsana in Sirsāsana – stage 4

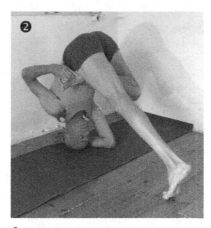

Ūrdhva Padmāsana in Sirsāsana – stage 2

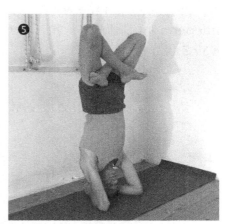

Ūrdhva Padmāsana in Sirsāsana – final stage

Sālamba Sirsāsana I

Variation 28 (Cont'd)
Learning Ūrdhva Padmāsana: Using the wall

II. Using internal wall corner

The corner provides a support that allows you to lift one hand at a time, and use it to improve the folding of the opposite leg:

→ Do *Sirsāsana* against an internal wall corner (see Variation 5 on page 18). Stand slightly away and equidistant from the two walls and lean the buttocks against them.

> Bend the right leg.

> Support yourself in the corner and use the left hand to arrange the right foot in its place for *Ardha Padmāsana* ❶.

> Then bend the left leg, this time use the right hand to move the left foot to the top of the right thigh ❷.

> Lift the knees up and move slightly away from the wall to do independent *Ūrdhva Padmāsana* in *Sirsāsana* ❸.

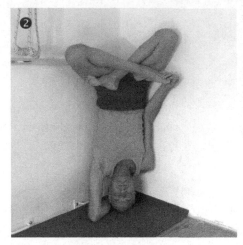

Ūrdhva Padmāsana in *Sirsāsana* – using internal corner - stage 2

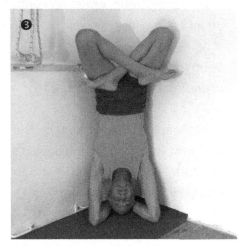

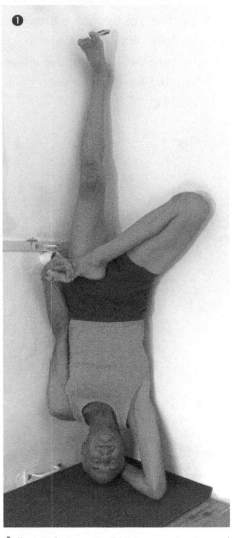

Ūrdhva Padmāsana in *Sirsāsana* – using internal corner - stage 1

Ūrdhva Padmāsana in *Sirsāsana* – using internal corner - final stage

Sālamba Sirsāsana

Variation 29
Advanced Sirsāsana variations: Back to the wall

Effects

The wall helps to keep the balance when learning to move the hands to the more advanced variations of Sirsāsana. These variations give firmness and confidence in balance.

Props

wall

This Variation is for advanced practitioners who wish to learn the additional hand positions of *Sirsāsana*. The wall helps to learn to move the arms swiftly from *Sirsāsana I*, to *Sirsāsana II* (LOY Pl. 192), *Sirsāsana III* (LOY Pl. 194), *Baddha Hasta Sirsāsana* (LOY Pl. 198) and *Mukta Hasta Sirsāsana* (LOY Pl. 201).

> **Note:** Advanced practitioners can stay in *Sālamba Sirsāsana I* for 20 minutes or more; however, I do not recommend staying more than a minute or two in each of the following *Sirsāsana* variations, as this may place an excessive load on the neck.

→ Do *Sirsāsana I* with your back against the wall (the knuckles and heels should touch the wall).

› Supporting the heels against the wall, move both arms quickly to *Sirsāsana II* ❶. Keep the hands and elbows at shoulder distance. Press the palms down to lift the shoulders.

› Move the arms back to *Sirsāsana I*. Repeat several times moving to *Sirsāsana II* and back, until you feel comfortable.

› Then move to *Sirsāsana III* ❷ and from there continue in the same manner to the other variations ❸&❹.

❶

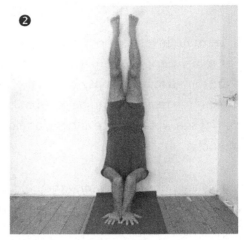

Sirsāsana II – back to the wall

❷

Sirsāsana III – back to the wall

❸

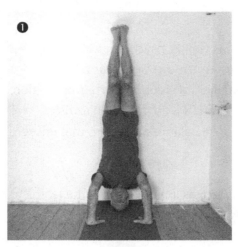

Baddha Hasta Sirsāsana – back to the wall

❹

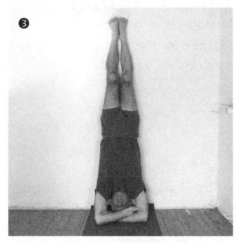

Mukta Hasta Sirsāsana - back to the wall

T i p s

✔ The key for keeping balance while switching the arm positions is to maintain a perfect vertical alignment on the crown of the head before you move.

✔ Move from one variation to another by shifting both arms quickly and concurrently.

✔ In *Sirsāsana II* keep the arms parallel to each other. Also, keep the forearms perpendicular to the floor and the upper arms parallel to the floor.

✔ In *Sirsāsana III*, spread the legs slightly to avoid losing the balance.

✔ After getting confidence with the wall support in this way, try to do these variations away from the wall. You can also try to go up to *Sirsāsana II* directly from *Prasārita Pādōttānāsana*.

Sālamba Sirsāsana

Variation 30
Advanced Sirsāsana variations:
Facing the wall

Effects

Doing Sirsāsana facing the wall has a peculiar effect: the eyes become soft and stable; since the eyes are connected to the brain, this makes the brain quiet.

Placing the toes against the wall helps to keep the balance when shifting from Sirsāsana I to Sirsāsana II and to the other advanced variations of Sirsāsana.

Props

wall

In learning inversions one faces physical as well as psychological challenges. For many people, the psychological barrier is more significant. We are not accustomed to being topsy-turvy, where our field of vision is inverted. In addition, there is the fear of falling back. What is behind us is an unknown territory – we do not see what is there and are afraid to lose balance and roll to that unseen, unknown space.

In this Variation of *Sirsāsana* the field of vision is limited; hence one learns to face unfamiliar states and accept them with confidence and equanimity.

There are several ways to enter the pose and to come out of it. I show here a simple way, in which you end up doing the pose at about 40 cm (16 inches) away from the wall. It is possible to do the pose closer to the wall, even with the elbows almost touching it, but entering the pose may be challenging, so I leave it to you to explore how to do the pose closer to the wall.

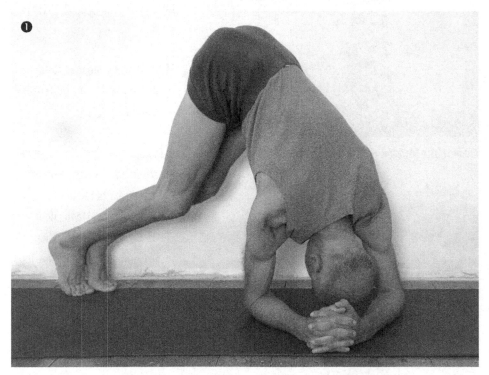

❶

Entering *Sirsāsana* facing the wall

➡️ Kneel with your side to the wall and place the forearms and the cup-shaped palms in front of the wall, such that your elbows are about 40 cm (16 inches) away from the wall ❶.

❯ Press the forearms down to lift the shoulders and stabilize the neck and head, then lift your legs and place the toes against the wall ❷.

❯ Straighten the legs and climb up the wall ❸.

❯ In the pose: Widen your gaze and stay without focusing on any specific point, but with soft and internalized (but open) eyes. Observe the effect of having the wall in front of you.

❯ After a few minutes, place the tips of the toes against the wall and using that support, move the arms to *Sirsāsana II* ❹.

❯ Press the palms down, balance and move the toes away from the wall. Stay for about a minute ❺.

❯ In the same manner do *Sirsāsana III* (LOY Pl. 194) and *Baddha Hasta Sirsāsana* (LOY Pl. 198) (not shown).

❯ Come out of the pose by turning sideways, as in ❶. Then stay for a while in *Adho Mukha Vīrāsana*.

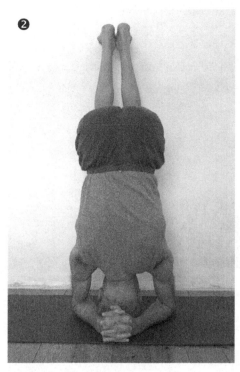

❷

Facing the wall – climbing up

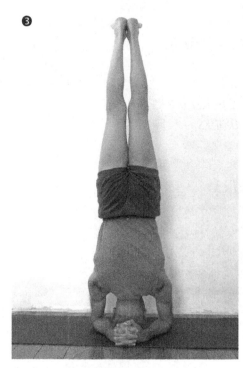

❸

Sirsāsana I - facing the wall

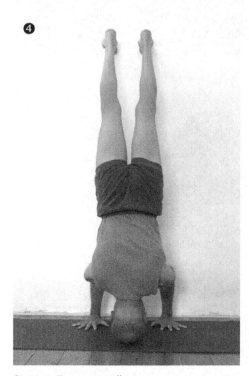

❹

Sirsāsana II - toes on wall

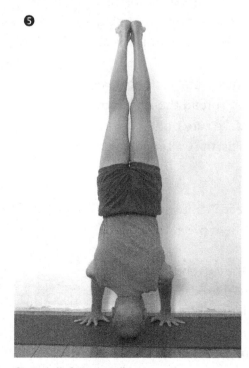

❺

Sirsāsana II - facing a wall

Doing *Sirsāsana* when there are Neck Problems

In some cases, it is impossible and even dangerous to do independent *Sirsāsana*. Examples are herniated or injured cervical vertebrae, injury in the skull, and severe stiffness in the upper back or shoulders. Luckily, Guruji Iyengar developed various ways that enable people who suffer from such symptoms to do the pose with props and enjoy its tremendous benefits.

Sālamba Sirsāsana I

Variation 31
Supporting the upper back: Using rods or planks

Effects
The rods support the trapezius muscle and/or the shoulder blades and hence reduce to a large extent the load on the neck

Props
2 metal or wooden rods, optional: chair

> ⚠ **WARNING**
> Do this Variation only under the guidance of an experienced Iyengar Yoga teacher. Do not attempt it if you have a serious neck injury or deformation.

A pair of rods or bars leaning on the wall or on a chair can be used to lift and support the trapezius muscles. This way the head is almost hanging and there is no pressure on the neck.

→ Lean two metal rods against the wall and spread their bottom edges ❶. Make sure both rods are leaning against the wall at the same angle.

❯ Place the head in between the rods and move them closer to the neck.

❯ Straighten the legs and step forward until you feel the rods are supporting the shoulder girdle ❷.

❯ Then lift the legs one by one to go up to the pose ❸.

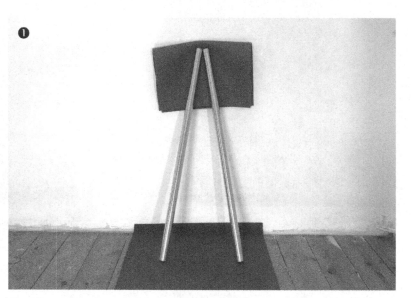

❶

Placing rods on the wall

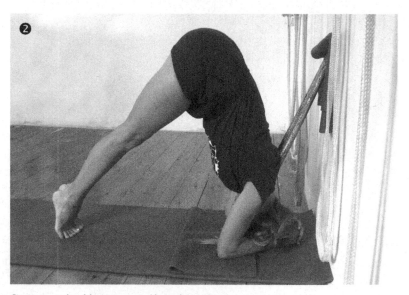

❷

Sirsāsana – shoulders supported by rods – stage 1

Sālamba Sirsāsana I

Variation 31 (Cont'd)
Supporting the upper back:
Using rods or planks

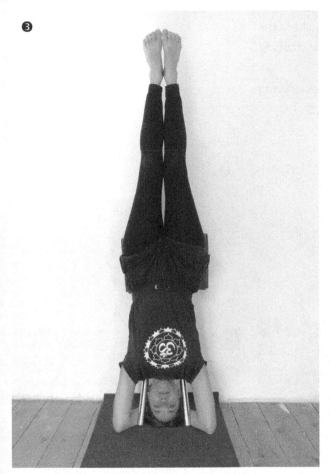

Sirsāsana – shoulders supported by rods – final stage

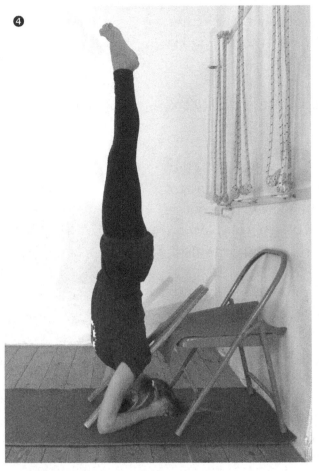

Sirsāsana - shoulders supported by planks on a chair

Notes:

1. If the ends of the rods are not equipped with rubber caps, place a piece of sticky mat between the rods and the wall to prevent slippage.

2. If the head is floating in the air while in the pose, you can place a 3-folded blanket under it.

3. You can also use two identical wooden planks/rods instead of metal rods.

4. Instead of leaning the rods on wall, you can lean them on the seat of a chair. Photo ❹ shows this with flat wooden planks.

Tips

✔ If you feel that the pressure on your two shoulders is uneven: check if the rods are leaning against the wall at the same angle.

✔ Experiment and find out which angle is most adequate to the structure and flexibility of your shoulder girdle. More vertical rods support the shoulder blades better, whereas more horizontal rods support the upper trapezius better.

Sālamba Sirsāsana I

Variation 32
Hanging the head:
Using two chairs

Effects

The chairs enable one to do the pose without any load on the neck. Hung in between the two chairs the neck is completely released. Still, unlike rope Sirsāsana, the pose is active, since you need to press the shoulders down and stretch the legs up.

Props

2 chairs, 2 rolled mats, wall

⟶ Spread a sticky mat next to the wall and place on it two chairs facing each other.

〉 Roll two sticky mats and place one on each seat.

> **Note:** Roll the mats so that they have equal diameter and density. Another option is to place a foam block on each chair (not shown).

〉 The distance between the two chairs should allow the head to enter between them.

〉 Stand in front of the chairs, bend forward; move the head down in between the chairs and rest the shoulders on the rolled mats. The backs of the shoulders should be supported by the wall.

〉 Now, gently draw the chairs closer to each other and to the neck. The rolled mats should touch the sides of the neck (to support the inner trapezius) ❶.

〉 As an intermediate stage you can place the knees on the chairs ❷.

〉 Press the palms on the chair to lift the legs up.

〉 Place the heels against the wall and stay in the pose.

> Keep lifting yourself by pushing the shoulders down against the chairs ❸.

> If you feel balanced, try placing your upper arms on the seats ❹.

❶
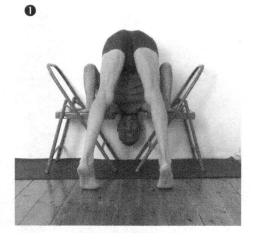
Entering *Sirsāsana* in between two chairs

❷
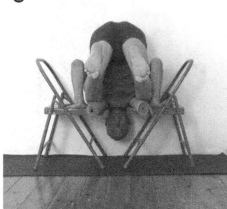
Lifting the knees to the chairs

❸
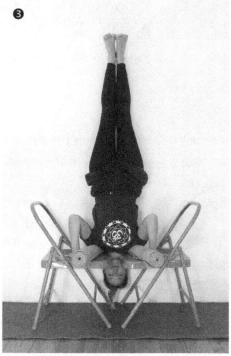
Sirsāsana on 2 chairs

❹
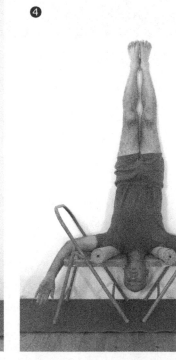
Sirsāsana on 2 chairs – arms resting sideways

An alternative to chairs

⟶ Make two stacks of 7 foam blocks and place the stacks next to the wall.

❯ Come up to *Sirsāsana*, like when doing with two chairs ❶.

There are also special *Sirsāsana* props that enable one to support the entire weight of the body on the shoulders such that the neck and head hang freely. Photos ❷ & ❸ show the usage of such a prop.

❷

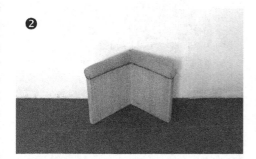

A special '*Sirsāsana* prop'

❶

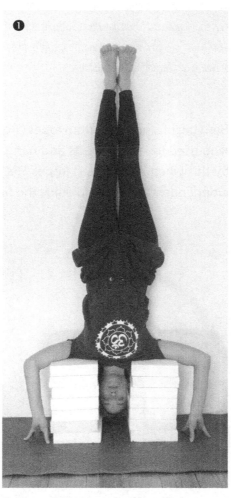

Sirsāsana - Using two stacks of foam blocks

❸

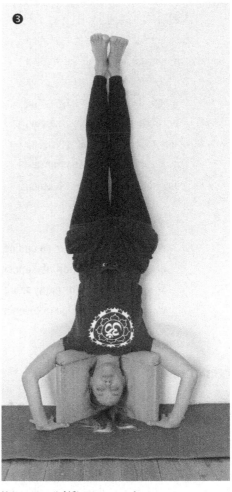

Using a special '*Sirsāsana* prop'

Sālamba Sirsāsana I

Variation 33
Restorative Sirsāsana:
Hanging from ropes

> ⚠ **CAUTIONS**
>
> Do not attempt this Variation without guidance and supervision of an experienced Iyengar Yoga teacher. The method of tying the rope and the correct positioning of the rope around your pelvis are critical for your safety and must be learnt from an Iyengar Yoga teacher!

Effects

Hanging in Sirsāsana enables people with injured necks, or those who cannot support their body weight using the arms and shoulders, to enjoy many of the benefits of this invaluable āsana.

This is a very relaxing way of being upside-down. Gravity extends the spine, releases compression of the vertebrae and expands the inner body cavities, thus enabling deep and soft breathing. With practice, you can easily stay more than 10 minutes on the rope and use this special condition for deep breathing as well as contemplation and meditation.

Props

two ropes anchored to top hooks ('top ropes'), another unanchored rope for tying, a few blankets, belt (optional)

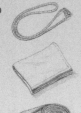

Hanging upside-down from ropes ('Ropes-*Sirsāsana*') mimics the ancient Yogis, who used to live in forests and hang from trees. Guruji Iyengar was inspired by this when he invented Ropes-*Sirsāsana* to enable people who cannot do independent *Sirsāsana* to enjoy the benefits of the "king of all *āsana-s*."

Note: Here I just give an outline of the basic variation of Ropes-*Sirsāsana*; there are many more variations, which I plan to cover in a future book.

Preparations:

→ Insert the unanchored rope in a top rope (make a lasso loop around it) ❶.

❯ Tie the knot-side of the unanchored rope to the adjacent top rope ❷. Make sure the knot is secured.

❯ Place two blankets on the rope for cushioning the buttocks and the sides of the hips.

Note: It is also possible to wrap a blanket around your hips and tighten it with a belt (like a skirt) ❸.

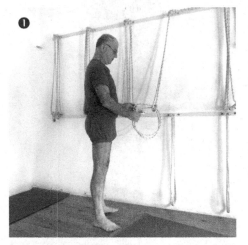

Inserting a rope for *Sirsāsana*

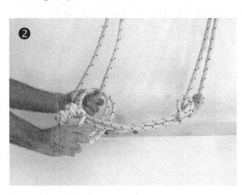

Tying rope for *Sirsāsana*

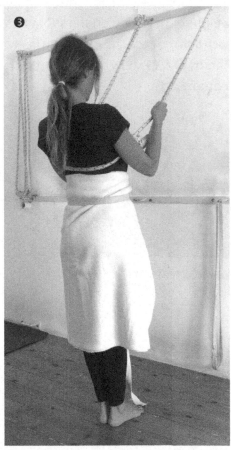

Rope *Sirsāsana* – stage 1

Sālamba Sirsāsana I

Variation 33 (Cont'd)
Restorative Sirsāsana:
Hanging from ropes

Going into the pose:

⟶ Stand facing the wall with the rope behind you and hold it against the sacral band.

❯ Climb on the wall and press your feet against the wall ❹ (you may support your heels by the two middle hooks).

❯ Adjust the rope to make sure it is on the sacral band.

> ***Note:*** At this stage, it is possible to place a folded blanket on the front thighs to have more cushioning.

❯ Hold the two top ropes, bend the legs and widen the knees between the two top ropes and the wall.

❯ Now the legs and the bottom rope hold your body weight; bend your legs and rest the body fully on the bottom rope.

❯ Join the feet as in *Baddha Koṇāsana* and move them in front of the top ropes ❺, or rest them on the wall.

❯ Release the arms down or interlock them at the elbows.

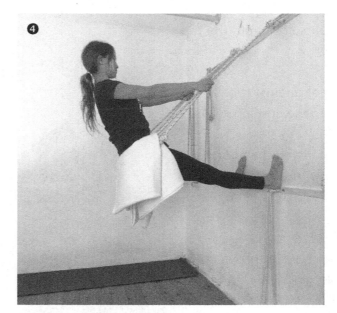

Standing on the wall to adjust the rope

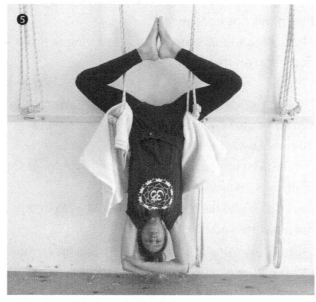

Sirsāsana - hanging from wall ropes

Variation 33 (Cont'd)
Restorative Sirsāsana:
Hanging from ropes

Coming out of the pose:

→ Lift yourself to hold the top ropes.

❯ Push the feet against the wall to come back to the position of ❹.

❯ Go down; stand on the floor. Keep the arms over the ropes and lean the forehead on the wall ❻.

> *Note:* Keeping the arms over the ropes is safer since it protects from losing the balance due to dizziness which may sometimes occur when coming out from the pose.

❯ Stay for a while in this position, and then go to *Adho Mukha Vīrāsana*, placing the forehead on the floor.

> *Note:* After being upside-down for an extended time, you should come out of the pose slowly and lean on the wall. Inhale while coming up from the upside-down position to prevent dizziness. This allows the blood pressure to adjust to the change.

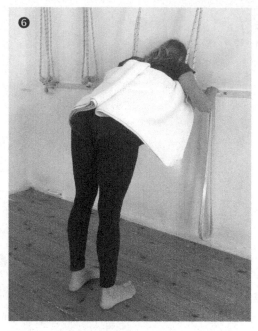

❻

Coming out of Rope *Sirsāsana*

Tips

✓ It is tempting to replace active *Sirsāsana* with Ropes-*Sirsāsana*. However, remember that active *Sirsāsana* has many physiological and psychological benefits that cannot be attained by hanging passively from ropes. Personally, I practice both independent and hanging *Sirsāsana* on a daily basis, and find that the effects are quite different, though, in a way, complementary and supplementary.

Referring to Rope *Sirsāsana* Guruji Iyengar had said in an interview:

> *"When we do Sālamba Sirsāsana on the ropes, our brain becomes empty like animals in sleep. Animals can remain immobile for a long time… Like a gorilla hangs from a tree, I do Sālamba Sirsāsana on the rope. It makes one's brain very passive and breathing becomes automatically slow, deep with unconscious retentions in between."*

But he also mentions that:

> *"this way I deadened my brain like a log of wood – insensitive."*[19]

[19] *Astadala Yoga Mala* Vol. 5 p. 109

Sālamba Sarvāngāsana and Cycle

As explained in the introduction for this chapter, *Sarvāngāsana* and its cycle is complementary to *Sirsāsana* and its cycle, and is usually practiced after it.

In the Iyengar Yoga method *Sarvāngāsana* and its cycle is done with the shoulders and upper arms raised on a platform, while the head rests on the floor. The platform should be long and wide enough to support the shoulders and the elbows; a platform of 50x50 cm (20x20 inches) is sufficient. The height should be about 5 cm (2 inches). For the type of blankets shown here, 5 to 6 blankets usually provide sufficient height; however, this may vary according to the type of blankets you use and the structure of your shoulder girdle. Try several different options and study the effects. You can also make a platform using four flat foam blocks and one or two blankets on top, or any other material that provides sufficient support.

In *Sarvāngāsana* and *Halāsana* the field of vision is limited and hence it is difficult to know if the body is properly aligned. For example, you may not notice that the two shoulders are not parallel to the platform's edge; or, that in *Halāsana*, the extended legs are not aligned with the centerline of the body. So I start with an explanation of a basic setup that helps to check and correct the alignment in *Sarvāngāsana*. Subsequent Variations teach the actions needed for this cycle and enable you to stay longer in the poses. Also included are restorative Variations which enable people with minor problems in the cervical spine to enjoy the benefit of *Sarvāngāsana*, and ideas on how to practice the *Sarvāngāsana* cycle when the props available are limited (like when traveling).

Sālamba Sarvāngāsana and Cycle

Variation 1
Basic arrangement for the
Sarvāngāsana cycle:
Using platform, bolster and block

Effects

The platform protects the neck and enables one to lift the upper back and to open the chest. The block and the bolster enable one to check and correct the alignment of the limbs in Halāsana. Once the base in Halāsana is correct, it can be maintained when going up to Sarvāngāsana. The bolster helps to lift the body into the pose and to roll down when you come out of it.

Props

4-7 blankets, belt, block, bolster (optional)

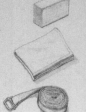

Why use a platform?

In Iyengar yoga, most props are used diversely, with a purpose to emphasize a certain action or effect. However, a platform for *Sarvāngāsana* is used consistently. Many students wonder about this, especially if they have practiced *Sarvāngāsana* without props in other yoga methods.

Using the platform has a basic anatomical explanation: the human anatomy does not allow the head to bend forward to form a 90° angle between the thoracic and the cervical spine. Photo ❶ shows bending the head forward from an upright sitting position.

If you insist on bending the head until the back of the skull is parallel to the floor, you necessarily have to curve the upper back ❷. This means that in *Sarvāngāsana* you will not be able to raise the thoracic spine and open the chest, and you will experience heavy load on the neck which may lead to injury. The platform is a simple and useful way to do an effective and safe *Sarvāngāsana*.

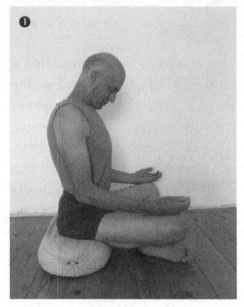
❶

It is impossible to stay upright and bend the head to 90°

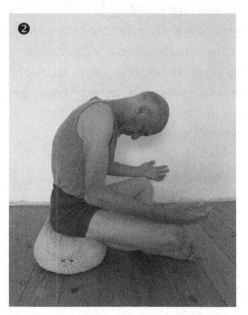
❷

A further bending necessarily curves the upper back

In this basic Variation I show how to use a platform to support the shoulders and the upper arms in *Sarvāngāsana* and *Halāsana*.

Preparation:

→ Place a bolster lengthwise in the middle of a mat.

❯ For head cushioning spread a 2-folded blanket on the mat. This allows the head to slide so that the neck will not contract.

❯ Stack several folded blankets on top of the spread blanket next to the bolster in order to create the platform.

Note: The height of the platform should be around 5 cm (2 inches).

❯ Align the rounded edges of the blankets to form a unified, smooth edge (on which the base of the neck will be supported) ❶.

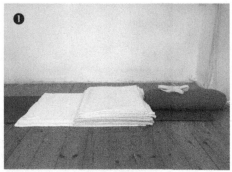
❶

Setup for *Sarvāngāsana* cycle

> Place a block lengthwise on the centerline of the mat. This block will support your toes in *Halāsana*. Measure the distance between the platform and the block as shown in ❷. Make sure that the centerlines of the block, the platform, the bolster and the mat are aligned. To prevent the block from sliding, place it on the mat.

> Adjust a belt to the width of your outer shoulders and place it near the platform.

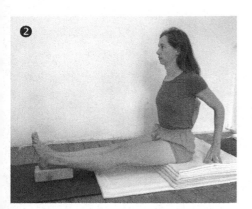

Measuring the distance between the platform and the block

Doing the cycle:

⟶ Lie with your upper back on the platform and pelvis on the bolster, spine in the center of the platform, such that the lower third of the neck is supported on the platform and the back of the head is on the cushioned mat. Leave a gap of about 3 fingers wide between the top shoulders and the edge of the platform.

> Make sure that both shoulders are equidistant from the edge of the platform and that the center of your body is aligned with the center of the mat (hold the edges of the mat to verify that).

> Lift your legs and roll over the head to *Halāsana*. Your toes should land on the block. If this is not the case, correct by moving the legs until you feel the toes resting on the center of the block ❸.

> Place the belt on the elbows.

> Interlock the fingers, move the shoulders back and roll the outer shoulders down, one by one, until you rest on the top of the shoulders. Make sure your neck is relaxed and can stretch freely away from the platform. If needed adjust the distance of the shoulders from the platform edge.

>> *Note:* This step is critical – do not go up to *Sarvāngāsana* before adjusting yourself on the top of the shoulders.

> Stretch the arms back along the sides of the bolster. Check that both arms are positioned evenly in relation to the bolster.

Now the arms and legs should be aligned symmetrically, in line with the centerline of the platform and mat.

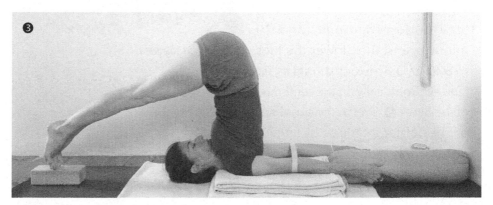

Halāsana with toes on block

Variation 1 (Cont'd)
*Basics arrangement for the
Sarvāngāsana cycle:
Using platform, bolster and block*

> Now fold the forearms to support the back with the palms. The fingers should face the spine and the thumbs support the sides ❹. Press down the upper arms and use the palms to lift the back ribs and open the chest.

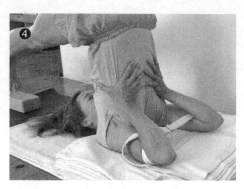

Palms position for *Sarvāngāsana*

> > *T i p s*
> > ✔ Join the tips of the middle or little fingers to verify that both palms are placed symmetrically around the spine and support the back at the same height ❹.

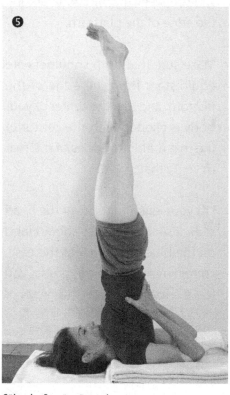

> Lift the legs (one by one or both together) and stretch up to *Sālamba Sarvāngāsana I* ❺.

> > *T i p s*
> > ✔ Stretch the legs up and lift the back from the upper back to the buttocks.
> >
> > ✔ Tighten the mid-buttocks in, and move the front thighs up and back.

Sālamba Sarvāngāsana I

> Stay in *Sarvāngāsana* for 5-10 minutes, and then lower the legs to *Halāsana*. The toes should again land symmetrically on the centerline of the block ❸. Stretch the arms back on the bolster, interlock the fingers.

> Stay in *Halāsana* for 3-5 minutes.

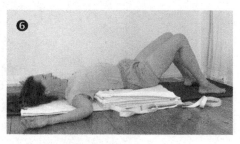

Coming out of *Sarvāngāsana*

> To get out of the pose, remove the belt off the arms, support the back with the palms and slowly roll the back to the platform, until the pelvis rests on the bolster.

> Slide from the platform to the head side until the shoulders rest on the floor, but the chest is still on the platform. You can bend the legs and rest for a minute or so ❻, before rolling to the right and coming out of the pose.

> *T i p s* for *Halāsana*
> ✔ Look up to verify that the two legs meet above the centerline of your face.
>
> ✔ Move the shoulders inward, i.e. toward each other to support yourself on the outer shoulder.
>
> ✔ Move the upper back forward until the top of the chest touches the chin.

Variation 2
Finding the alignment in Sālamba Sarvāngāsana

It is both important and challenging to find the correct alignment in the pose. Ask a teacher or a friend to verify the following points (see also: *Astadala Yoga Mala* Vol. 6 Plate n. 9).

Looking from the front observe that:

- Both shoulders are at the same distance from the edge of the platform (a)

- The lower third of the back of the neck is supported, and the upper part is free (not on the platform) (b)

- The head is centered and is not tilted left or right (c)

- The body is aligned symmetrically about its longitudinal midline from the skull to the feet (d).

- The midlines of both legs are facing forward and the big toes are joined (e)

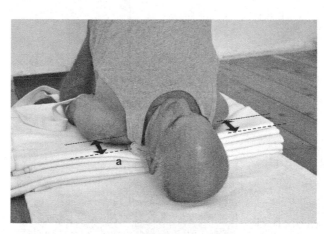

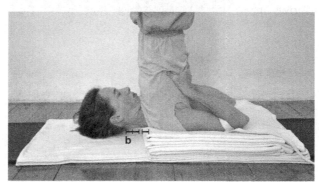

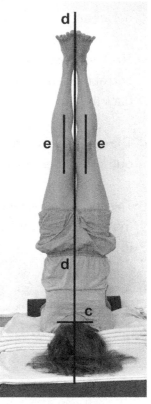

Observing *Sarvāngāsana* from the front

Variation 2 (Cont'd)
Finding the alignment in Sālamba Sarvāngāsana

Looking from the back observe that:

- The centerline of the body is vertical and divides the body to two even halves (a)

- The hands are placed symmetrically and at the same height on the mid-back (b)

- The outer elbows are in line with the outer shoulders (c)

- The upper arms extend straight back (not diagonally) and the elbows are in line (d)

Looking from the side observe that:

- The center of the armpit is vertically aligned with the hip joint and the ankles, and this midline divides the body evenly between the front and the rear sides (a)

- The spine is straight and the upper back is not rounded (b)

- The buttocks are lifted (c)

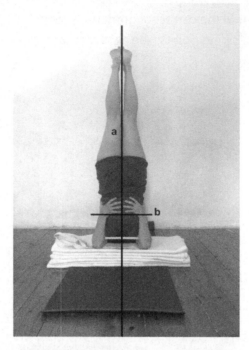

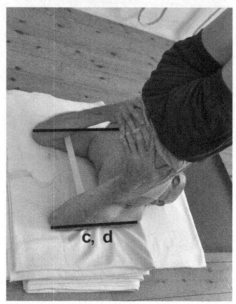

Observing *Sarvāngāsana* from the back

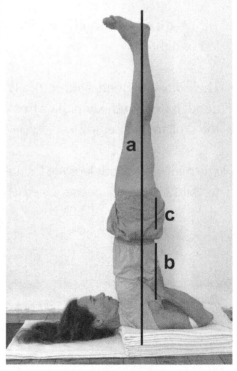

Observing *Sarvāngāsana* from the side

Effects

The plank provides grounding for the elbows and helps to support the back,
which in turn helps to open the chest.

Props

5-7 blankets, belt,
plank or extra mat

In *Sarvāngāsana* the body weight is
borne by the shoulders, upper arms
and elbows. If the shoulders are stiff,
the elbows cannot reach the platform
and the body weight is borne by the
muscle power of the arms and back
rather than by the bones. This may
be tiresome and stressful. Adding
support under the elbows enables you
to transfer load to the arm bones, even
when the shoulders are stiff.

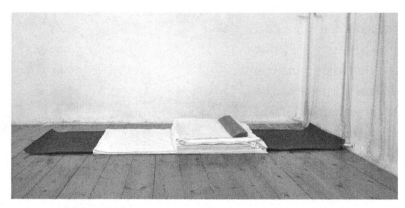

Placing a plank for the elbows

→ Prepare the platform as usual
and place a plank on its rear side,
such that the narrow side of the
plank is toward the front of the
platform.

> **Note:** A folded mat can be used
instead of the plank.

> Go to *Halāsana* and adjust the
position of the plank such that it
supports the upper arms, just above
the elbows.

> Place the belt on the elbows and
press the elbows down against the
plank to go up to *Sarvāngāsana*.

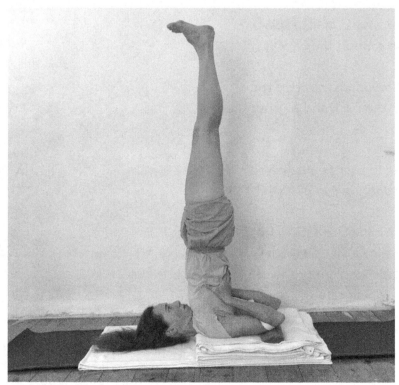

Sarvāngāsana with plank under elbows

T i p s

✔ Press the elbows directly downwards
and use the palms to make the back
ribs concave.

✔ Turn the biceps out and press down
the outer upper arms and outer
elbows.

Variation 4
Supporting the back with a plank

Effects

The plank helps to lift the upper back, push the shoulder blades in and open the chest. It also enables one to do the pose when, for some reason, the palms cannot be used to support the back.

Props

5-7 blankets, belt, plank

Some people find it difficult to support the back with the palms, usually due to stiffness in the shoulders or pain in the wrists. In such cases a plank can be used as a mediator between the palms and the back. You can try this Variation even if you can support the back with the palms, since it teaches the action required from the back muscles in order to open the chest.

➡️ Go to *Halāsana*, hold the plank and use it to support the back ❶.

❯ Go up to *Sarvāṅgāsana*. Use the plank to lift the back and to push the back ribs in ❷.

❯ It is possible to use the plank also for *Setu Bandha Sarvāṅgāsana* ❸.

Another option is to place a sticky mat piece on the palms. This is especially useful for people who tend to sweat excessively, in which case the palms slip on the back ❹.

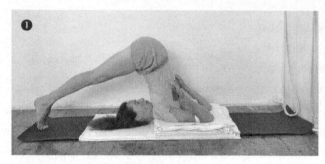

Placing the plank on the back in *Halāsana*

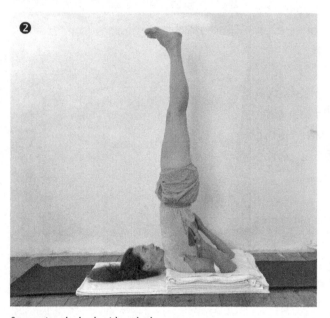

Supporting the back with a plank

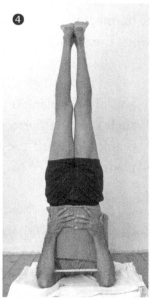

Placing a sticky mat piece on the back

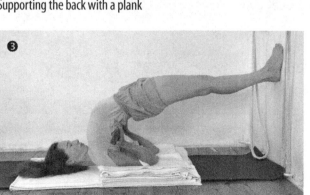

Setu Bandha Sarvāṅgāsana with plank

Tips

✔️ In order to lower the support toward the upper back, use a long plank and hold it wider than shoulder-width.

Sālamba Sarvāngāsana and Cycle

Variation 5
Moving the thoracic dorsal spine in:
Feet against wall

Effects

Pushing the wall with the feet helps to lift the upper back and to move the thoracic dorsal vertebrae in. It can also help people suffering from lower back pain in Sarvāngāsana, since it helps to activate the buttocks up toward the ceiling against the force of gravity, instead of resting heavily on the lower back.

Props

5-7 blankets, belt, wall

⟶ Prepare the platform such that the head-side is away from the wall, about 60 cm (2 feet) away from it.

❯ Climb on the wall to lift the back from the platform. Place the belt on the elbows.

❯ Bend the knees, place the feet on the wall and push against it to lift the upper back and to make it more concave.

❯ Stay in the pose, pushing against the wall and move the top chest to touch the chin.

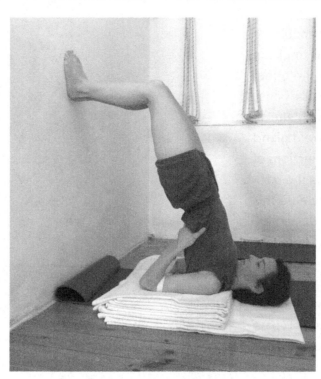

Sarvāngāsana - feet pushing against the wall

Tips
✔ Relax the back of the neck and the throat and allow the chin to roll toward the notch between the collar bones.

Variation 6
Improving the Jālandhara Bandha effect: Supporting the back of the head

Effects

Increased stimulation of the organs of the neck, including the thyroid. The back of the neck is extended without being compressed on the floor.

Props

5-7 blankets, belt, rolled bandage or towel

In *Sarvāngāsana* the chest should be lifted and moved forward until the manubrium (the top sternum bone) and the notch between the collar bones touch the chin. This has deep effects since it stimulates the thyroid gland which controls many vital functions of our body and it invigorates the back of the brain. In order to increase this effect, you can place a rolled bandage or towel under the occiput (the back of the skull).

→ Arrange the platform for *Sarvāngāsana* as usual and prepare a rolled bandage next to it.

❯ Go into *Halāsana*. Place the rolled bandage under the neck. Slide the roll toward the back of the skull while extending the back of the neck and rolling the head toward the chest.

❯ Lift the upper back and move the dorsal vertebrae in, until the top chest touches the chin. Then go up to *Sarvāngāsana*; keep lifting the chest to maintain the touch of the manubrium with the chin.

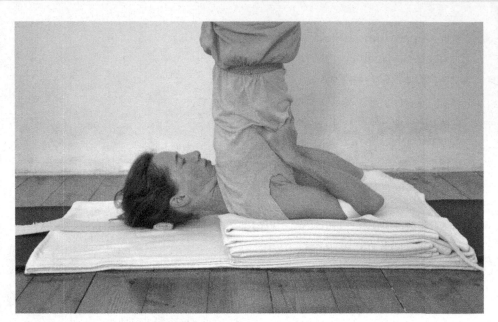

Sarvāngāsana with a bandage under the head

Tips

✓ Adjust the thickness of the roll according to your needs by partly unfolding the bandage.

Effects

The blankets support only the back of the neck, allowing the shoulders more freedom of movement. The chair is used to support the back (replacing the hands). These create more movement in the shoulders and more opening of the chest. The back is lifted and the chest is moved forward to create a deep Jālandhara Bandha effect.

Props

chair, several blankets, additional sticky mat (or sticky piece), wall (optional)

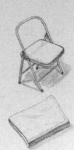

In this Variation a chair is used to create more movement in the shoulders and chest (and not for restorative purposes as shown in Variation 16, on page 85). The blankets are folded to a narrow platform and placed lengthwise to support the back of the neck; this enables one to insert the arms under the front rung of the chair (when there is one) and to move the shoulders further back.

⟶ Place the chair near the wall.

❯ Place a folded sticky mat (or a sticky piece) on the seat of the chair and place on top of it 1-3 folded blankets (to increase the height of the seat according to your needs).

❯ Fold 2-3 blankets to make a narrow platform and place this platform lengthwise under the chair, such that its edge protrudes about 20 cm (8 inches) from the front of the chair.

❯ Sit sideway on the chair and roll to lift the legs and lie on the chair with the feet supported on the wall.

❯ Hold the chair and pull yourself closer to the back of the chair.

❯ Insert the arms under the chair and hold the back legs of the chair. If the chair has a front rung, insert the arms under that rung, and not above it.

❯ Now slide down until the lower part of the neck is supported by the edge of the narrow platform ❶.

❯ Pull the shoulders back and if possible bend your arms over the front legs of the chair to increase the movement of the shoulders ❷.

❯ Try different ways of using the arms to create more movement in the shoulders ❸, ❹.

❯ Stay in the pose for 3-6 minutes. Then lower the legs to *Halāsana* ❺.

✔ **Tips** To prevent rolling sideways, spread the legs slightly.

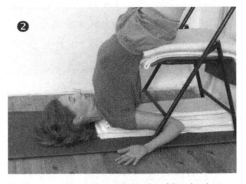

Bending the elbows to pull the shoulders back

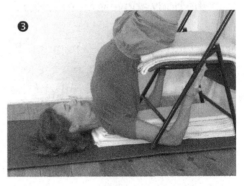

Pressing the forearms against the legs of the chair

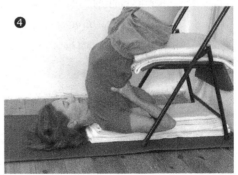

Supporting the back to make it concave

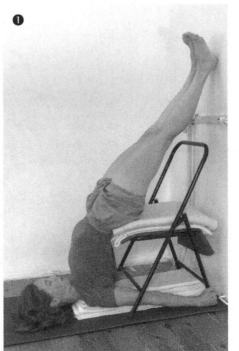

"Chair *Sarvāngāsana*" with arms under the rung

Variation 7 (Cont'd)
Active "Chair Sarvāṅgāsana":
Using a chair to support the back

> Stay in *Halāsana* for a few minutes, and then pull the chair toward you, until the front edge of the seat touches your back.

> Hold firmly the legs of the chair and pull it toward you to support the back as you lift your legs up to *Sarvāṅgāsana* ❻. Adjust your grip to maintain the vertical alignment of the body above your shoulders.

> Stay in the pose for 3-6 minutes. To come out of the pose move the legs backward, release the grip of the chair and slide down to rest your back on the floor.

T i p s

✔ When placing the blankets on the chair, let them hang slightly over the front of the seat, in order to cushion its contact with your back.

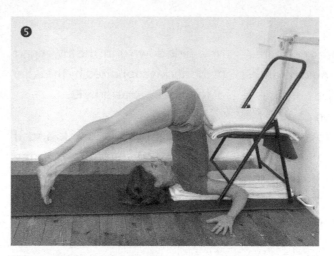

❺

Halāsana with legs slightly spread

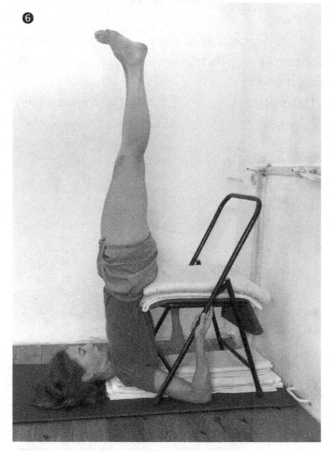

❻

Active *Sarvāṅgāsana* with chair supporting the back

Props

5-6 blankets, belt,
bolster, metal rod
(optional)

In *Sālamba Sarvāngāsana II* (LOY Pl. 235) the palms are not used to support the back. It is still a *sā-lamba* (with support) pose, but the support is achieved by pressing the arms and hands down against the floor. Usually, the platform is not long enough to support the wrists and hands, and this weakens the base of the pose. An additional support can alleviate this problem. We use a bolster next to the platform.

Here are two ways to support the hands in order to improve the base of the pose:

I. <u>A belt on the wrists</u> ❶ – To make the arms firmer you can shorten the belt as shown in Variation 3 of *Halāsana* on page 90.

II. <u>Holding a rod</u> ❷ – The rod should be heavy (about 10 Kg or 22 lbs.). (See also Variation 4 of *Halāsana* on page 91).

The improved stability of the wrists and arms enables one to lift the back better.

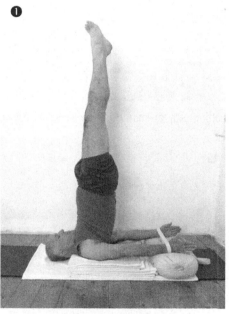

Sālamba Sarvāngāsana II with belt on the wrists

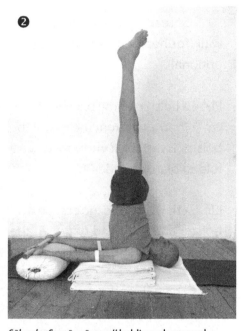

Sālamba Sarvāngāsana II holding a heavy rod

T i p s

✔ You can move dynamically several times from *Halāsana* to *Sālamba Sarvāngāsana II* and back, each time increasing the pressure of the arms down as you lift the legs. Try to keep the legs straight and joined and move them slowly with exalation.

Variation 9
*Nirālamba Sarvāngāsana:
Facing the wall*

Effects

Climbing up the wall helps to lift the back and to make it more concave. The support of the wall teaches one to balance on the shoulders in Nirālamba Sarvāngāsana II (LOY Pl. 237). The wall also helps to spread the legs further in Supta Koṇāsana.

Props

bolster, wall,
optional: 2 blankets,
belt, another bolster

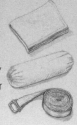

In this Variation *Sarvāngāsana* is done facing the wall with the toes against the wall. The *Supta Koṇāsana* variation is especially beneficial here, since the wall aids in increasing the stretch of the inner legs.

→ Spread a blanket next to the wall (for head cushioning – this is optional).

❯ Place a bolster on the blanket, 30-40 cm (1 foot) away from the wall. If the bolster is not thick enough, place a folded blanket under it.

❯ Lie with your shoulders on the bolster and the head between the wall and the bolster ❶.

❯ Press the hands down and roll up toward the wall; bend the knees and place them against the wall ❷.

> ***Note:*** It is recommended to place another bolster lengthwise under the back to facilitate the rolling into the pose.

❯ Stretch the arms back, interlock the fingers and pull the shoulders back to position them on the centerline of the bolster.

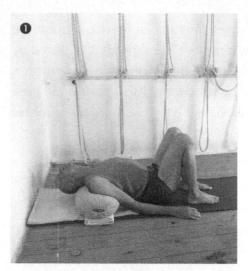
Getting ready to climb up to *Nirālamba Sarvāngāsana*

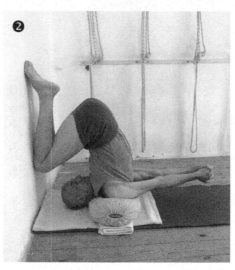
Positioning the shoulders for *Nirālamba Sarvāngāsana*

❯ Now press the palms against the wall and climb with toes up the wall. Use the support of the toes and hands against the wall, to lift the back and make it concave ❸.

❯ In order to balance, slowly move the toes away from the wall and stretch the legs vertically up. Then remove the hands from the wall and stretch the arms up along the body, palms facing away from the wall. Stay for a few minutes with normal breathing ❹.

❯ Then spread the legs and lower them down to *Supta Koṇāsana*. Press the feet against the wall, catch the feet and stretch the legs ❺.

❯ You can also do *Karnapidāsana* with the back of the feet on the wall (not shown).

If you wish to combine *Sālamba Sarvāngāsana* with *Nirālamba Sarvāngāsana*, use another bolster and a belt for elbows support. After using the wall to lift the back, you may experience a better *Sālamba Sarvāngāsana* ❻.

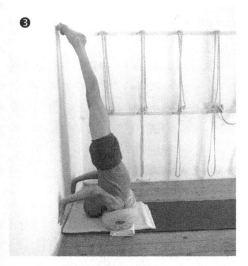

③

Using the wall to lift the back

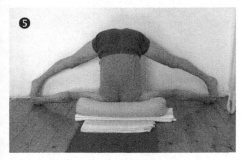

⑤

Supta Koṇāsana - feet against the wall

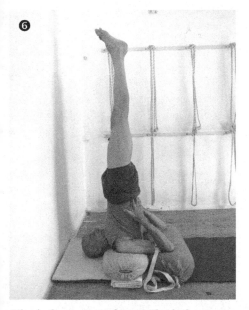

⑥

Sālamba Sarvāngāsana from *Nirālamba Sarvāngāsana*

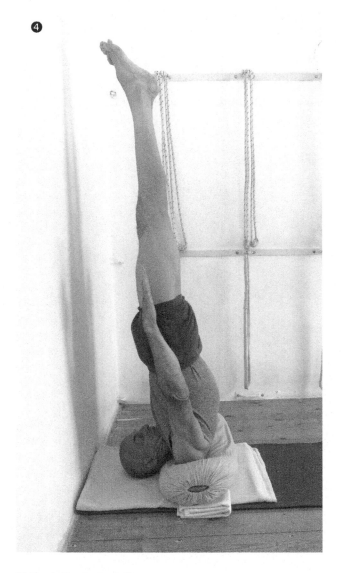

④

Nirālamba Sarvāngāsana II

Doing *Sarvāngāsana* when there are neck problems

In *Astadala Yoga Mala*, Guruji Iyengar wrote:

> *"In my years of practice and teaching I came across numbers of people who got pains in their necks. I devised ways of performing this āsana without pain."*[20]

And indeed, Guruji Iyengar had invented ways to do *Sālamba Sarvāngāsana* even when there are neck injuries.

 CAUTIONS

Doing *Sarvāngāsana* when there is a cervical spine disc protrusion is risky. If you suspect you have this condition consult a knowledgeable certified Iyengar Yoga teacher.

---

[20] *Astadala Yoga Mala* Vol. 6, p. 308

Sālamba Sarvāngāsana and Cycle

Variation 10
*Doing the pose when C7 is protruding:
A platform for each shoulder*

Effects
This Variation enables one to do Sarvāngāsana even when the base of the neck is protruding and sore.

Props
7 blankets, belt

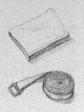

Imagine doing *Sarvāngāsana* on a platform which is weight sensitive, such that it becomes darker where there is more weight. What should be the pattern on such a platform after doing *Sarvāngāsana* on it? Ideally the body weight should be borne on the shoulders and upper arms only. The back of the neck, including vertebrae T1 and C7 should be lifted off the platform. Hence, such a platform should show two parallel dark lines, each reflecting an upper arm - from the shoulder to the corresponding elbow.

When the base of the cervical spine (vertebra C7) is protruding, doing classic *Sarvāngāsana* may be painful. This Variation enables those who suffer from this condition to do the pose without pain.

→ Prepare two small platforms; each from 2-3 folded blankets (fold them one more fold compared with the regular platform).

> Place the two platforms with the round edges facing each other, leaving a small gap in between for the cervical spine ❶.

> Lie down on your back such that each shoulder rests on its corresponding platform and the base of the cervical spine is between the two platforms.

> Go up to *Sarvāngāsana* ❷.

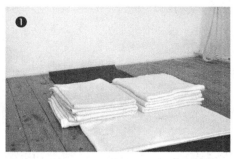

Two platforms with a small gap in between

> Push the shoulders down and attempt to lift the spine, especially vertebrae T1 and C7.

Tips

✔ Before going up to the pose, make sure to move the shoulders in (toward each other) and roll the outer shoulders down. Support yourself on the heads (tops) of the shoulders and not on the upper back.

✔ In the pose, keep pressing the outer shoulders and outer elbows down and stretch the legs up to lift the entire spine.

Note: This Variation can be performed on a standard *Sarvāngāsana* platform. Simply add two folded blankets along the centerline of the platform ❸.

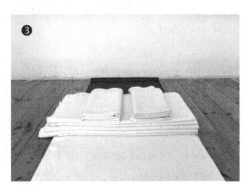

Sarvāngāsana on two platforms

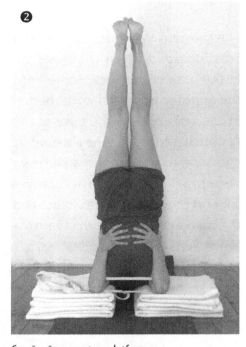

Adding two folded blankets on the platform

Sālamba Sarvāṅgāsana and Cycle

Variation 11
Lifting the neck and spine:
Supporting the neck with a lengthwise blanket

Effects

The folded blanket supports the base of the neck and helps to lift the spine upward. This, combined with other āsana-s that curve the neck, helps to correct the deformity of the C7 protrusion.

Props

5-7 blankets, belt

The previous Variation allows doing *Sarvāṅgāsana* when there is pain at the base of the neck. Sometimes the opposite approach works better: instead of allowing the base of the neck to hang freely in the air, support it in order to lift the entire spine from vertebra T1 upward. The blanket support provides a soft resistance and directional input to lift and curve in the other direction.

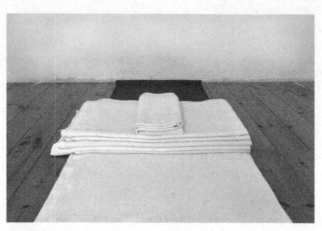

Additional blanket to support the cervical spine

⟶ Prepare the platform for *Sarvāṅgāsana* as usual.

❯ Take an additional 3-folded blanket and place it lengthwise in the middle of the platform.

❯ Go up to *Sarvāṅgāsana*. Use the additional support to lift the entire spine further up.

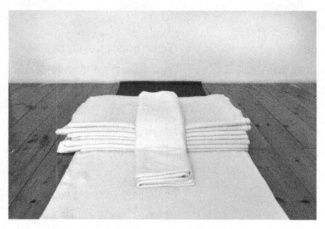

Supporting the cervical spine and the back of the head

Another option is to have the 3-folded blanket end extends slightly beyond the head side of the platform.

Tips

✔ Compare this Variation with the previous one to find out which helps you more to lift the spine. Remember that in a well-performed *Sarvāṅgāsana* the weight should be on the outer shoulders, outer upper arms and elbows – no vertebra should touch the platform.

Sālamba Sarvāngāsana and Cycle

Variation 12
Supporting the trapezius:
Using two rolls

Effects

The rolls lift the trapezius on both sides of the neck. This helps to free the shoulders, open the chest and lift the entire body up while preventing pressure, and possibly pain, in the neck. It can also help to correct a bulging C7 vertebra.

Props

5-7 blankets, belt, 2 rolled bandages

In *Sarvāngāsana* the trapezius muscle should be lifted up; in order to do so you need to roll the shoulders back and inward, until you rest on the outer shoulders. These actions are difficult to do when the trapezius muscle is stiff. In such cases the neck may be compressed and pain may be felt. If one is not careful, it can even injure the neck. In this Variation, the two rolls support the trapezius muscles.

> Prepare the platform for *Sarvāngāsana* as usual, and place the two rolled bandages on its front edge ❶.

> Lie on the platform; place the inner trapezius of each side of the neck, on a bandage.

> Go to *Halāsana* and readjust the bandages such that they support the top of the trapezius on both sides, close to the neck. The base of the neck (C7 vertebra) will be then slightly lifted.

> Place the belt on the elbows and go up to *Sarvāngāsana* ❷.

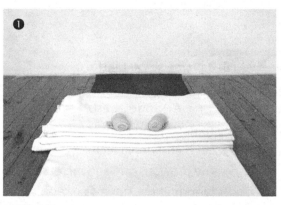

Position of bandages

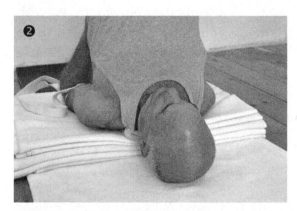

Sarvāngāsana with 2 bandages to support the trapezius muscle

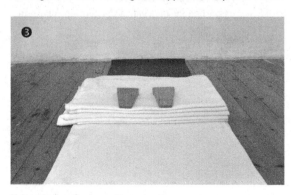

Using wedges for trapezius support

Note: The pressure of the bandages may cause pain, but this is not harmful, so if you can endure the pain - relax and let the trapezius muscles soften - the pain may go away. If the pain persists (or it is unbearable) make the roll thinner, by partly unfolding the bandages.

You can also use for this purpose two wooden wedges ❸, two thin metal cylinders (those used for knee treatment – not shown here), or other suitable material.

Sālamba Sarvāngāsana and Cycle

Variation 13
Supporting the neck:
Stepped-edge platform

Effects

When the neck muscles are tensed, having the neck hanging in the air may be painful. The slanted stepped edge of the platform fully supports the neck thus providing soft cushioning for it. This Variation is especially needed for people with inverted neck curvature (no lordosis or even kyphosis at the cervical). The rounded convex shape of the edge creates a healthy support for neck. In addition, the higher platform provides more freedom for the shoulder girdle and the upper back.

Props

7-8 blankets, belt

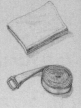

This Variation is useful when there is a minor pain or sensitivity in the neck region. Two ways to create the slanted edge of the platform are presented.

I. Stepped-Edge platform

⟶ Prepare a platform from 6-8 blankets (rather than 5). Build it such that the head side of the platform steps down toward the floor.

❯ Lie on the platform such that the back of the neck rests fully on the stepped edge of the platform ❶.

❯ Place the belt on the elbows and go to *Halāsana*, arrange the shoulders and go up to *Sarvāngāsana* ❷.

> *T i p s*
> ✔ Arrange the stepped edge of the platform to form a rounded (convex) slope in order to match the concave shape of the cervical spine (or to create it).
>
> ✔ If a *Simhāsana* box is available, you can use its sloping edge instead of the stepped platform.

II. Reverse slope platform

⟶ Arrange the blankets such that, starting from the 3ʳᵈ blanket, each additional blanket overhangs the previous one and increases the length of the slope ❸.

❯ Do *Sālamba Sarvāngāsana* with your neck on the reverse slope platform ❹.

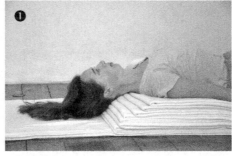

Supporting the neck with a stepped edge platform

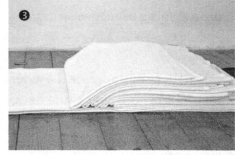

Supporting the neck with a reverse slope arrangement

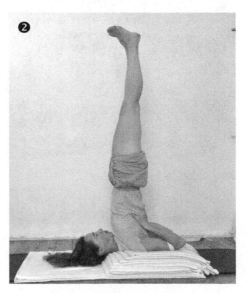

Sarvāngāsana on a stepped edge platform

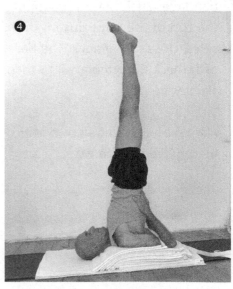

Sarvāngāsana with a reverse slope

Variation 14
*Supporting the neck:
platform of two bolsters*

Effects

Bolsters are thicker and softer than a standard platform (made of 5-6 blankets); hence they are more comfortable and enable doing the pose even when the neck is sensitive or the shoulders are very stiff.

Props

2 bolsters, blanket (optional), belt

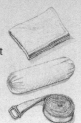

A bolsters-platform is comfortable and is useful when the neck is sore or the shoulders are stiff. However, the bolsters lack the stability and resistance that the blankets provide, from which to press the upper arms and elbows against. Also the higher support reduces the *Jālandhara Bandha* effect of the pose (which is created when the upper chest is in contact with the chin).

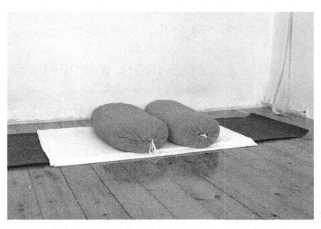

Using two bolsters as a platform

⟶ Spread a blanket and place on it two (even size) bolsters next to each other. One bolster serves for shoulders support and the other for elbows support. The blanket should extend beyond the head-side bolster so as to soften the contact between the head and the floor.

❯ Lie on the bolsters such that the shoulders rest on the centerline of the front bolster and the neck is fully supported by the rounded edge of that bolster.

❯ Go to *Halāsana*. Place the belt on the elbows and go up to the *Sarvāngāsana*.

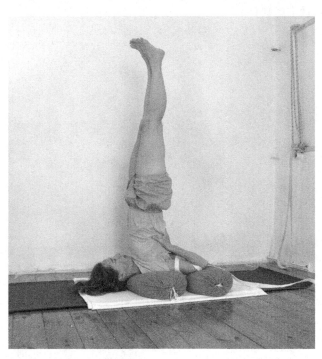

Sarvāngāsana on two bolsters

T i p s ....

✔ When using bolsters, support the entire back of the neck on the platform (rather than just the lower third as in a platform made of blankets). ......

Variation 15
Sarvāngāsana away from home:
Doing the pose with limited props

Here are three options to practice *Sarvāngāsana* with limited props.

Option 1: With 2 blankets

If only two blankets are available, you can make a reasonable platform by 3-folding each blanket. You get two strips, one for the shoulders and one for the elbows (the height of each strip is the same as that of a platform made of three blankets). This gives a reasonably good support for the shoulders and elbows ❶.

Option 2: Two blankets and two blocks

If you have blocks, you can use them to support the elbows ❷. The strip made from the two blankets is then sufficient (equal to platform made of six blankets).

Option 3: Four blocks

Blocks can also be used to support the shoulders ❸.

> **T i p s**
> ✔ If you use wooden blocks, you may place a folded sticky on them for cushioning

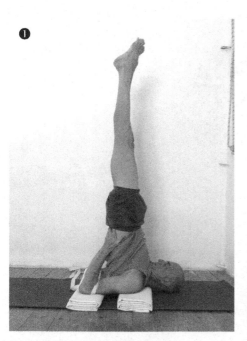

Sarvāngāsana on two 3-folded blankets

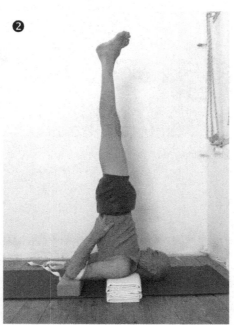

Sarvāngāsana on two 3-folded blankets and two blocks

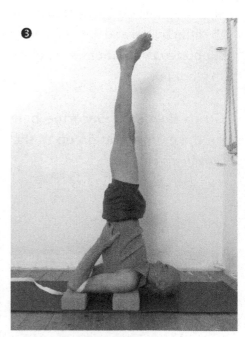

Sarvāngāsana on 4 blocks

When I travel I always take with me a thin sticky mat and two belts. If I have more space I take a light rubber block. But carrying 4-5 blankets in your suitcase is usually not possible, so doing *Sarvāngāsana* away from home is challenging. How then can one practice *Sarvāngāsana* in such situations?

This is when one needs creativity! Guruji Iyengar's development of the prop system is an example of great creativity. We can follow this example and use the lack of traditional props in these situations to be innovative in our environment. Obviously with the idea that while the use of regulated props is ideal, we should not halt our practice because of this obstacle!

Sarvāngāsana in a hotel room

In most hotel rooms there are blankets (not always the most appropriate ones, but still useable). If no proper blankets are available, use the sofa, pillows and any fabric available to improvise *Sarvāngāsana* and *Viparīta Karaṇi* as shown in ❶, ❷& ❸ and *Setu Bandha Sarvāngāsana* (not shown).

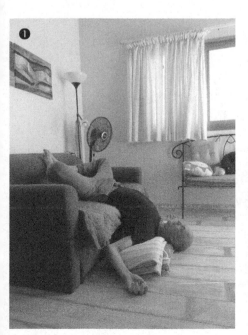

Viparīta Karaṇi - Baddha Konāsana variation

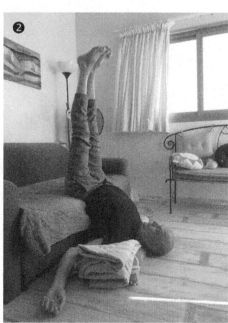

Viparīta Karaṇi

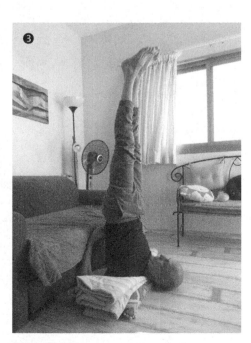

Sarvāngāsana

Variation 15 (Cont'd)
Sarvāngāsana away from home:
Doing the pose with limited props

My house is close to the Mediterranean beach, and for me the beach is a great place to practice. The Elements of Water (Ap) and Air (Vayu) fill me with energy. I have a quiet spot with some shade. I take to the beach only a towel and a belt – this does not prevent me from doing Sarvāngāsana!

Sarvāngāsana on the beach

The sand can be formed to substitute various props. In *Sarvāngāsana*, instead of lifting the shoulders, it is easier and more stable to dig a shallow pit for the head ❶ (with some experience one learns the size and depth of this pit). This has further advantages since when going to *Halāsana* ❸ the feet are at shoulder level (instead of being lower). The same holds true for *Setu Bandha Sarvāngāsana* ❹ – when arching back you do not need to drop the feet lower than the level of the shoulders. This makes the pose easier and more natural.

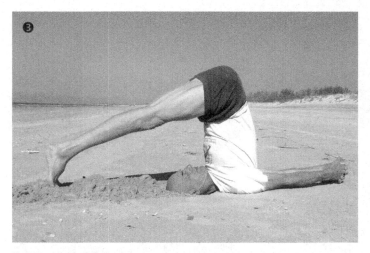

Preparing a pit in the sand for the head

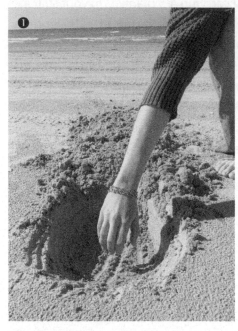

Sarvāngāsana on the beach – head is in a small pit

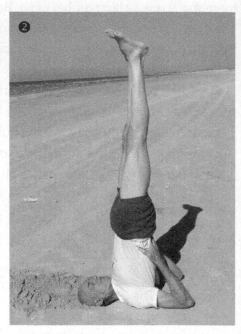

Halāsana on the beach

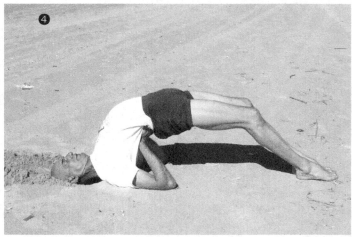

Dropping back to *Setu Bandha Sarvāngāsana*

Restorative Sarvāngāsana

Sālamba Sarvāngāsana and Cycle

Variation 16
Chair Sarvāngāsana

Effects

This is a very relaxing way to do Sarvāngāsana. People suffering from minor neck injuries or have very stiff shoulders, can still do the pose using a chair and enjoy its tremendous benefits. The support makes the pose very recuperative, since the lower body (buttocks and legs) does not need to be as active as in regular Sarvāngāsana. The chest is opened and deep breathing becomes natural; hence it is a good preparation for Prānāyāma.

Props

chair, bolster, sticky mat piece, 2-3 blankets, wall (optional)

There are several ways to use a chair for *Sarvāngāsana* (See: *A Chair for Yoga* by the same author and *Yoga in Action – Preliminary Course* P. 113 by Geeta Iyengar). We already saw how to use a chair in order to support the back in active *Sarvāngāsana* (see Variation 7 on page 71). Here I show the most common variation of using the chair for restorative *Sarvāngāsana*.

→ Place a chair next to the wall, with its backrest slightly (a few inches) away from the wall.

Note: The pose can be done without a wall, but if the seat of the chair is not high, then the legs tend to be more horizontal. Supporting the feet on a wall, allows the legs to be more vertical.

> Depending on your height and that of the chair, place 1 to 3 folded blankets on top of a sticky mat on the seat.

> Spread a blanket in front of the chair (to cushion the back of the head) and place a bolster in parallel to the front of the chair.

> Sit sideways on the chair, and then while holding the backrest roll on the buttocks to face the wall while lifting the legs up ❶.

> Bend the lower legs over the backrest (this stage is especially useful when doing the pose with no wall support) ❷.

> Then straighten the legs up the wall and pull yourself toward the wall until the buttocks are close to the wall ❸.

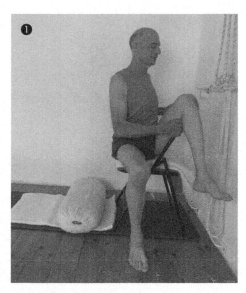

Entering Chair *Sarvāngāsana*

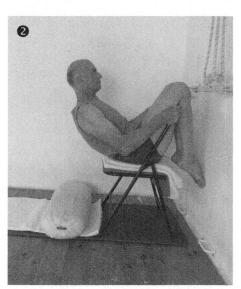

Bending the lower legs over the backrest (useful when doing the pose with no wall support)

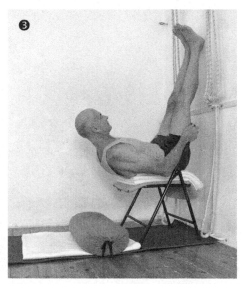

Chair *Sarvāngāsana* – pulling toward the back of the chair

Variation 16 (Cont'd)
Chair Sarvāngāsana

> Now you are lying safely on the chair, so release the backrest, and insert the arms under the seat (in between the front legs of the chair) and grip the back legs of the chair ❹.

> Slowly slide down and rest the shoulders on the centerline of the bolster. Keep the waist held on the seat of the chair.

> Hold the back horizontal rung of the chair with the palms facing up.

> Grip the hands on the rung firmly to lift and expand the chest and to pull the shoulders back until the back of the neck rests freely on the rounded edge of the bolster. Your weight should be distributed between the chair and the bolster ❺.

Note: if holding the back rung is too challenging for your shoulders, or if your arms are long, hold the back legs of the chair.

> Stay in the *āsana* from 5 to 10 minutes; breathe slowly and deeply and keep the brain passive.

> To come out of the pose, loosen the grip of the chair and gradually slide down until the buttocks are resting on the bolster. Wait in this position for a while before rolling sideways to sit up.

Leg positions

→ The legs can lean against the wall ❺ or stretch vertically up ❻ or fold into *Baddha Koṇāsana* ❼ or *Padmāsana* ❽.

Notes:

1. If the neck feels compressed (because the bolster is not thick enough), or the seat is too high for you, place a 3–folded blanket under the bolster to raise the shoulders more.

2. If the seat is too low, place a few additional folded blankets or a foam block on the seat to increase its height.

3. If the backrest is too high to support the feet for *Baddha Koṇāsana*, tighten a belt on the backrest ❾.

Doing variations

The chair can be used to do variations like *Pārśva Sarvāngāsana* (LOY Pl. 254) ❿, *Halāsana* ⓫, *Supta Koṇāsana* ⓬ and *Pārśva Halāsana* ⓭.

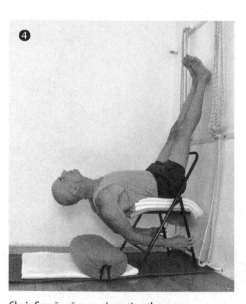
Chair *Sarvāngāsana* – inserting the arms

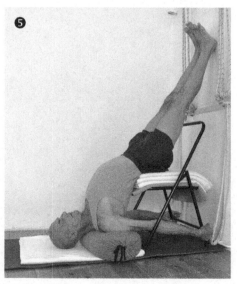
Chair *Sarvāngāsana* - legs on the wall

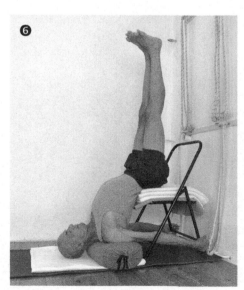
Chair *Sarvāngāsana* - legs stretched vertically

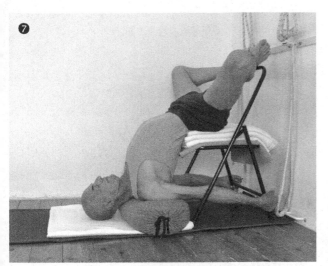

Chair *Sarvāngāsana* - legs folded in *Baddha Koṇāsana*

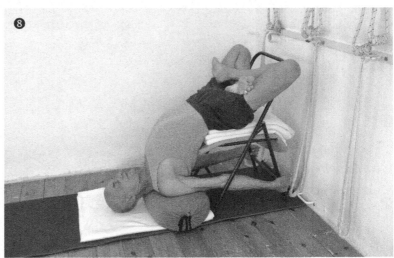

Chair *Sarvāngāsana* - legs in *Padmāsana*

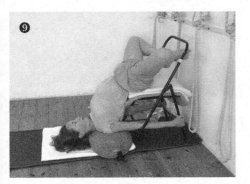

Using a belt for *Baddha Koṇāsana*

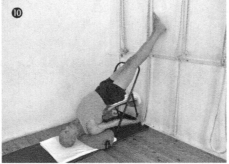

Pārśva Sarvāngāsana on chair, feet on wall

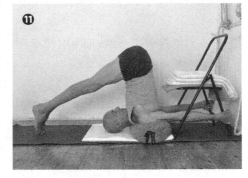

Halāsana – holding the chair

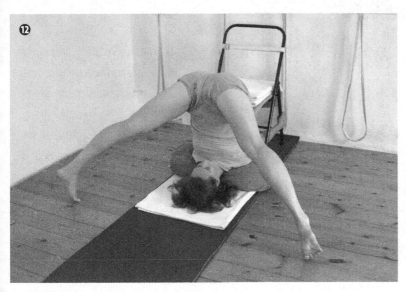

Supta Koṇāsana

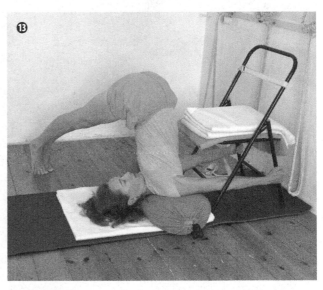

Pārśva Halāsana

Halāsana and other variations

Halāsana and other variations

Variation 1
*Supporting the legs to lift the back:
Toes on chair*

Effects
*The chair provides higher feet support for people who cannot reach the floor
with their toes. It also helps to position the shoulders correctly, to lift the trunk
and to move the thoracic vertebrae into the body.*

Props
5-7 blankets, belt,
chair or stool

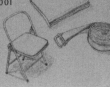

→ Prepare the standard platform
for *Sarvāngāsana* and place a chair
about 1 meter (3 feet) away from the
platform on the head side.

❯ Measure the distance of the chair
from the platform as in ❶ and move
it accordingly (if necessary).

❯ Go to *Halāsana* placing the tips of
the toes on the chair.

❯ Press the toes against the seat and
lift the thighs up ❷.

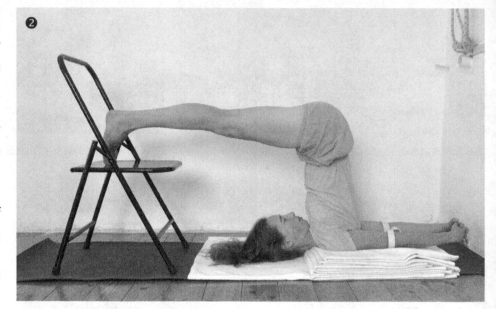

Halāsana – toes on chair

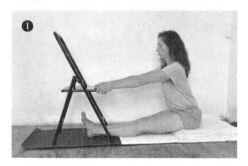

Measuring the distance of the chair

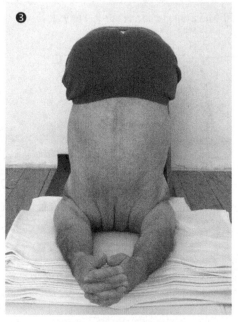

The spine forms a shallow canal along the center of
the back

Tips

✔ *Lift the hips vertically up; move the
thigh bones to the pelvis while rolling
the buttocks toward the heels.*

✔ *Move the thoracic dorsal spine into the
body and lift the entire trunk. When
this action is correct, the vertebrae sink
below the back muscles and the spine
forms a shallow canal along the center
of the back ❸.*

✔ *Lift the front thighs and open the backs
of the knees.*

Variation 2
Supta Koṇāsana: Toes on chairs

Effects

This Variation is similar to the previous one, but here the legs are spread apart. This helps to widen the lower back and the pelvis region.

Props

5-7 blankets (or 2 bolsters), 2 chairs

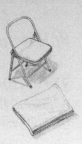

→ Prepare the standard platform for *Sarvāngāsana* or use a bolster to support the shoulders.

❯ Place the chairs diagonally, about 1 meter (3 feet) away from the platform on either side.

❯ Lie on the platform, roll up and spread the legs. Place the tips of the toes on the chairs.

❯ Press the toes against the chairs and lift the thighs up.

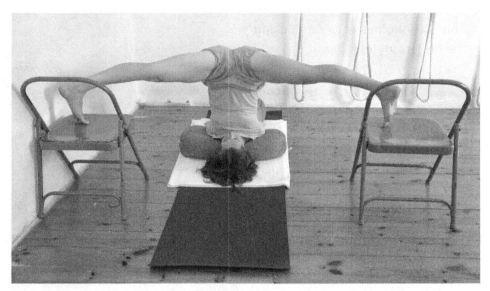

Supta Koṇāsana – toes on chairs

Variation 3
Adjusting the shoulders:
Belt on wrists

Effects

Working against the resistance of the belt activates the arms and helps to roll the shoulders back and down. People with stiff shoulders may find it hard to interlock the fingers in Halāsana; this variation is a good substitute for them.

Props
5-7 blankets, belt

This is an alternative to interlocking the fingers in *Halāsana*:

→ After coming down from *Sarvāngāsana*, remove the belt, shorten it and place it on the wrists.

❯ Turn the palms to face the ceiling.

T i p s

✔ Push against the belt and roll the outer shoulders further down toward the floor and toward each other.

✔ Press the arms down, move the shoulder blades in and up to open the chest.

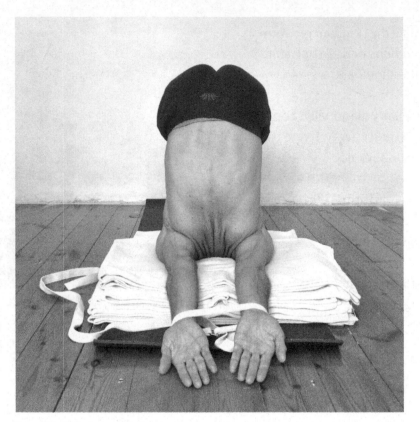

Using a small loop on wrists

Halāsana and other variations

Variation 4
Creating movement in stiff shoulders: Holding a rod

Effects

The weight of the rod helps to create movement in the shoulders and increases their flexibility. This is especially useful for people with stiffness in the shoulders. It also stabilizes the pose.

Props

5-7 blankets, heavy metal rod

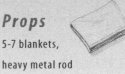

→ Place a heavy metal rod near the platform.

> **Note:** The weight of the rod should be 5 to 10 kg (10 to 20 lbs.), depending on the body's structure and flexibility.

> Go to *Halāsana* and catch the rod behind the back, with the palms facing up at shoulder width. Stretch the arms and press them down on the platform with the help of the rod ❶.

> Lift the front thighs and extend the back upward.

> The rod can also be used in *Sarvāngāsana* ❷.

> An alternative to this is to hold wall hooks located close to the floor ❸.

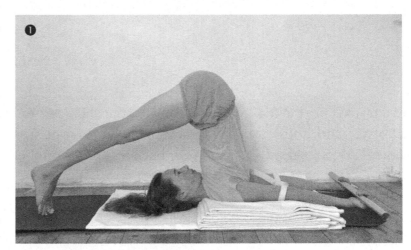

Holding a metal rod

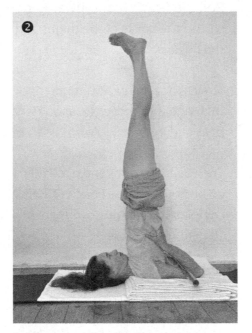

Sarvāngāsana with metal rod on arms

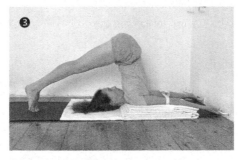

Holding lower wall hooks

Applicability:

All the Halāsana variations, especially Pārśva Halāsana.

Halāsana and other variations

Variation 5
Restorative Halāsana:
Thighs on bench (Ardha Halāsana)

Effects

This is one of the best restorative poses; you can relax deeply, and enter a tranquil, sublime and passive state of mind. The support for the thighs extends the lower back and hence this variation is very useful for people suffering from lower back problems. It is a good way to 'cool down' after a strong back-bending practice.

Props

2 bolsters, blanket, chair or bench (a 'Halāsana box') – the height of the bench should be about 50 to 60 cm (2 feet), depending on the length of your upper body and the height of the shoulders support.

➤ Spread a blanket next to the widthwise bolster and under a *Halāsana* bench.

➤ If necessary, place a sticky mat piece and a few blankets on top of the bench.

➤ Place two bolsters near the bench in a T shape; the widthwise bolster for shoulder support, and the lengthwise bolster to help in going into the pose and to soften the coming out of the pose ❶.

Notes:

1. If only one bolster is available, replace the lengthwise bolster with any suitable support.

2. Adjust the number of blankets on the bench according to your need.

3. If the neck feels compressed (because the bolster is not thick enough), or if the bench (or chair) is too high for you, place under the bolster a 3–folded blanket to raise the shoulders a bit more.

➤ Lie down with your shoulders on the center of the widthwise bolster and your back and pelvis on the lengthwise bolster.

➤ Roll and lift up to *Halāsana*, placing the thighs on the bench.

➤ Roll the front thighs inward and spread the backs of the thighs and the buttocks.

➤ Stretch the arms backward; interlock the fingers to move the shoulders back and in ❷.

➤ Then bend the arms and place them on both sides of the bench ❸. Relax completely in the pose; you can stay 10 minutes or more.

Note: In this pose, you may support either the upper thighs or the lower thighs and knees. The former is best for extending the lower back while the latter induces more softness in the lower back and the abdominal organs.

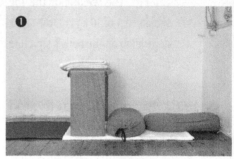

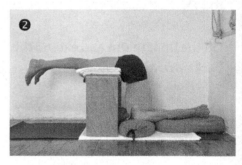

Arranging for restorative *Halāsana*

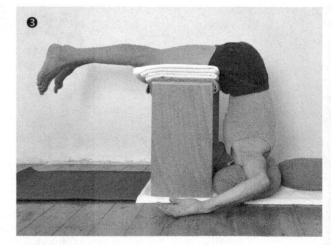

Ardha Halāsana with a bench – moving the shoulders back

Ardha *Halāsana* with a bench

Halāsana and other variations

Variation 5 (Cont'd)
Restorative Halāsana:
Thighs on bench (Ardha Halāsana)

The support for the knees is shown in ❹. You can either use a bench or a chair. Put a blanket (or a bolster) on the seat of the chair for cushioning or for adjusting the height according to your needs.

Another option that creates more space in the lower abdomen is to place a rolled sticky mat on the bench ❺.

If you can interlock your legs in *Padmāsana*, you can rest them on the bench ❻ – this is very effective, since it stretches the back farther and creates space in the abdominal organs.

When using a chair with low rungs, it may be impossible to insert the head under it. In this case use two chairs and place the head in between them ❼ & ❽.

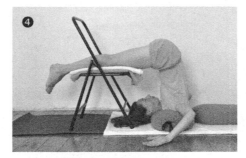
Ardha Halāsana with a chair

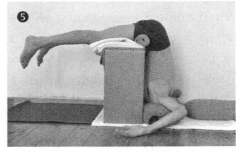
Ardha Halāsana – rolled mat under top thighs

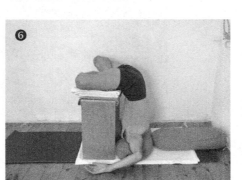
Padmāsana in *Ardha Halāsana*

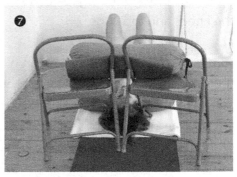
Ardha Halāsana on 2 chairs - preparation

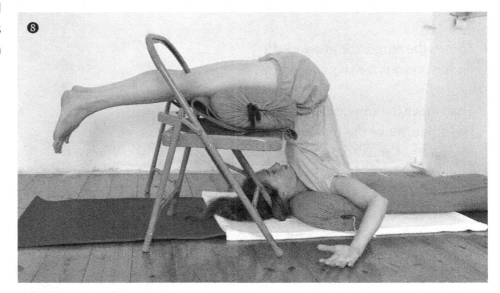
Ardha Halāsana on 2 chairs

Tips
✔ Use your exhalations to relax; exhale through the head and face (eyes, ears, cheeks, tongue, etc....).

Halāsana and other variations

Variation 6
Restorative Karnapidāsana:
Supporting the knees

Effects

Placing the knees on blocks (at the height of the platform or higher) provides support for the knees while touching the ears (as the name of the pose suggests). This is very relaxing!

Props

5-6 blankets or a
bolster, 2 blocks

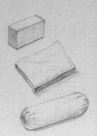

When doing *Karnapidāsana* on the floor, the knees rest on the floor, next to the ears. However, since in Iyengar Yoga we do *Sarvāngāsana* on a platform to protect the neck, when we proceed to *Karnapidāsana* the knees normally hang in the air (unless we collapse the pose to force them to the floor). The blocks fill the gap between the knees and the floor.

Karnapidāsana is usually done as part of the *Sarvāngāsana* cycle, in which case you have to prepare the two blocks in advance, and place them on either side of the mat, near the platform.

→ From *Halāsana*, bend the legs to *Karnapidāsana*.

❯ Stretch the arms back, interlock the fingers and pull the shoulders back.

❯ Then move the arms forward to the head side. Move the blocks closer to your head and rest the knees on them. Stay for 1-2 minutes.

> **Note:** If you are doing only *Halāsana* and *Karnapidāsana*, you can use a bolster to support the shoulders (instead of a platform made of blankets).

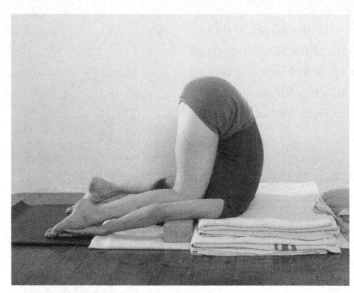

Karnapidāsana – knees on blocks

Setu Bandha Sarvāngāsana

About *Setu Bandha Sarvāngāsana*

Setu Bandha Sarvāngāsana is not really an inverted pose in the sense of being upside-down, but it is part of the *Sarvāngāsana* cycle; hence it is included here. It has a unique combination of a back bend in the chest region and a forward bend in the neck and head regions. The backbend opens the chest and charges the body with energy, but without over-activating and over-heating the brain. The head bows deeply towards the chest in a *Jālandhara Bandha*; this induces quietness, humbleness and inwardness. Hence, *Setu Bandha Sarvāngāsana* prepares well for *Śavāsana*.

In the *Sarvāngāsana* cycle one moves to *Setu Bandha Sarvāngāsana* by arching back and lowering the feet down to the floor. This lifts the thoracic spine, opens the chest and stretches the cervical spine – which releases the neck in case it was compressed while doing *Sarvāngāsana*. Arching back from *Sālamba Sarvāngāsana* all the way down to the floor is challenging for many practitioners. Doing this with props enables everyone to enjoy and benefit from it.

Setu Bandha Sarvāngāsana

Variation 1
Moving the Sacrum in:
Using a block

Effects

Placing the sacrum on the block moves it into the pelvis. The support of the block and the wall make the pose less demanding and one can stay for several minutes and enjoy its special effects. Tightening a belt around the thighs allows the legs to relax further.

Props

1 or 2 blocks, wall, belt (optional)

Place your mat perpendicular to the wall. Put one block next to the mat and the other one at the wall end of the mat.

> **Note:** The second block is optional and is used to support the heels. However, many people find it hard to do the pose without this support. This block can be placed lying on its side as shown, or standing.

> Lie on the back with feet on the wall at an appropriate distance and tighten a belt around the upper thighs (belt not shown here).

> **Tips**
> ✔ Get an estimate of the distance of the pelvis from the floor by lying on the back with feet placed on the wall, such that the legs are lifted to 30° from the floor ❶.

> Bend the knees and lift the pelvis (as if doing *Chatushpādāsana*), take the block and place it under the lower sacrum (the sacro-coccyx area).

> Rest the pelvis on the block and stretch the legs one by one to the wall. Push the feet against the wall and press the back-heel bones down against the second block ❸ or against the floor ❹. Move the front thighs down (toward the floor).

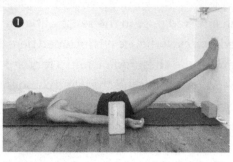

Measuring the distance to the wall for *Setu Bandha Sarvāngāsana* with block

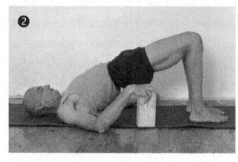

Inserting the block (lengthwise)

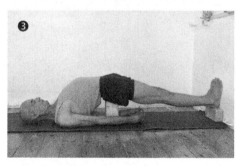

Setu Bandha Sarvāngāsana with block for sacrum and block for heels

> Interlock the fingers behind your back, pull the shoulders toward the wall and lift the chest up.

> **Tips**
> ✔ If possible, lower the legs down and move the front thighs back (toward the floor), this will lift and open the chest.

> ✔ The block supports the sacrum but not the back; engage the back muscles and lift the back ribs in order to open the chest.

> ✔ Breathe deeply to further open the top chest.

> After adjusting the shoulders you can release the fingers' interlock. Stay in the pose for 5-7 minutes, then bend the knees, lift the pelvis, move the block away, and rest with the back on the floor in *Dwi Pāda Supta Pavanamuktāsana* ❺.

> To release the back it is recommended to do *Adho Mukha Swastikāsana* with a block under the forehead ❻.

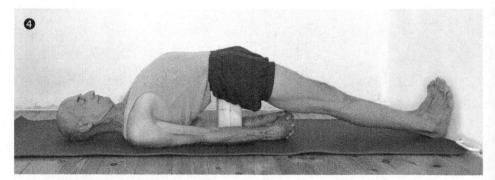

Setu Bandha Sarvāngāsana with block for sacrum

> After adjusting the shoulders you can release the fingers' interlock. Stay in the pose for 5-7 minutes, then bend the knees, lift the pelvis, move the block away, and rest with the back on the floor in *Dwi Pāda Supta Pavanamuktāsana*.

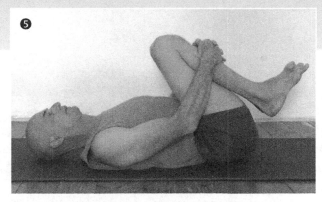

Releasing the lower back in *Dwi Pāda Supta Pavanamuktāsana*

> To release the back it is recommended to do *Adho Mukha Swastikāsana* with a block under the forehead.

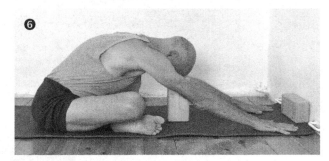

Releasing the back in *Adho Mukha Swastikāsana*

How to place the block?

The block can be placed on the sacrum lengthwise, as shown in ❶ or widthwise as shown in ❷ & ❸. In case of a lengthwise block, make sure not to place it under the lumbar (it may extend below the coccyx).

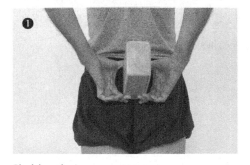

Block lengthwise

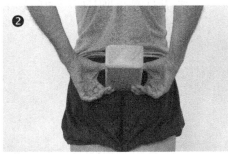

Block widthwise

> *T i p s*
> ✔ Compare these two options: lengthwise block creates a sharper action on the sacrum and the tailbone, while widthwise block is more soothing and less demanding.

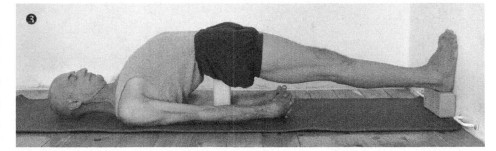

Using the block widthwise

Setu Bandha Sarvāṅgāsana

Variation 1 (Cont'd)
Moving the Sacrum in:
Using a block

Using higher support

Higher support for the sacrum opens the chest further. The standard size blocks are appropriate for most people, but advanced practitioners can use two blocks to get a higher support.

> Insert a highest-block on top of a lowest-height-block **❶**; or vice versa **❷**.

The second option gives wider support but requires balancing the top block on the narrow edge of the standing block.

> *T i p s*
> ✔ Make sure that your shoulders are resting on the floor, this is essential in order to get the relaxing effect of the pose. If necessary, place folded blankets under the shoulders and head.

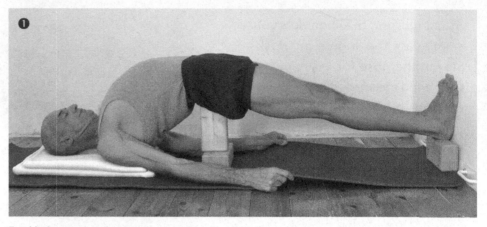

Two blocks: standing one on top

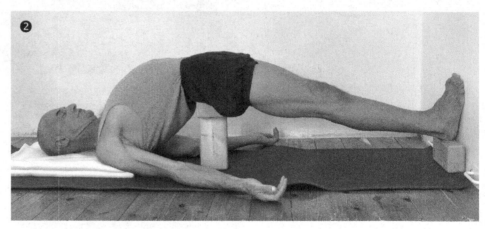

Two blocks: lower-height block on top

Setu Bandha Sarvāngāsana

Variation 2
A wider support:
Pelvis on two blocks

Effects

*The wider support and the lift of the sides, rather than the center, are soothing.
The abdominal organs soften and recede towards the lower back. The lower
abdomen is contained by the pelvis.*

Props

2 - 3 blocks, wall, belt

This Variation is similar to the previous one, but instead of using a single block to support the sacrum, two blocks are used to support the sides of the sacrum.

➡ Place two blocks next to your mat and prepare another block (optional) for the feet next to the wall.

❯ Place the blocks on either sides of the sacrum.

❯ Lie on the back at an appropriate distance from the wall and tighten a belt around the upper thighs.

❯ Bend the knees, lift the pelvis (as if doing *Chatushpādāsana*) and insert the blocks under the sides of the sacrum (the sacroiliacs).

❯ Do the pose as in the previous Variation.

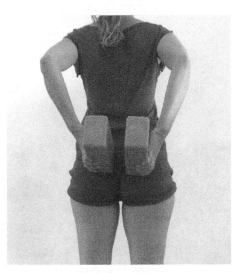

Placing two blocks for wider support

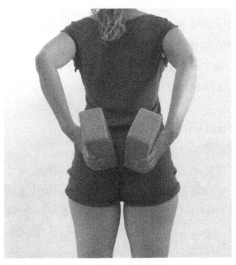

Placing the blocks in a triangular shape

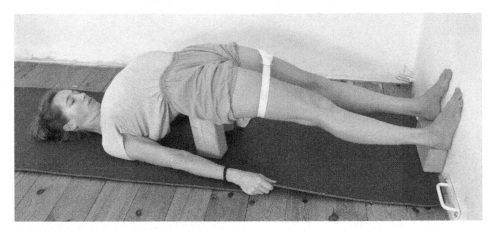

Setu Bandha Sarvāngāsana with wider block support

Tips

✔ Experiment to find out which arrangement of the two blocks gives you the best support. Try to adjust the blocks in a triangular fashion with the narrow side of the triangle supporting the sacrococcyx (sacrococcygeal symphysis).

✔ The blocks should support the hips as if to form a cradle shape in the lower abdomen. Soften the navel region and allow it to recede toward the lower back and to move up toward the chest.

Setu Bandha Sarvāngāsana

Variation 3
Opening the chest:
Helper pulls the shoulder blades

Effects
The pull of the rope increases the opening of the chest and the top of the lungs for full breathing. The pressure on the shoulders descends the tops of the shoulders to the floor. This creates an exhilarating feeling combined with relaxation.

Props
belt or rope, 2 blocks, helper, blanket (optional)

This Variation is a continuation of the two previous ones, but the opening of the chest is increased when a helper pulls the shoulder blades.

Student:

⟶ Do *Setu Bandha Sarvāngāsana* with a block supporting the sacrum, as described in Variation 1 or 2 above. Before lying down, place the rope on the floor under your shoulder blades.

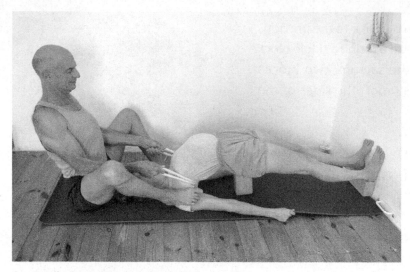

Setu Bandha Sarvāngāsana - helper pulls shoulder blades

Helper:

⟶ Separate the two sides of the rope's loop and place the lower strip on the lower part of the student's shoulder blades and the other strip on the upper part of the shoulder blades.

❯ Place your feet gently against the student's shoulders.

> **Note:** Match the rounded shape of the student's shoulders with the concave shape of the arches of your feet.

❯ Pull the belt while pressing your feet gently against the student's shoulders.

❯ Keep pulling the belt diagonally upward to lift the student's chest.

T i p s

✔ **Helper:** If the student experiences too much stretch at the back of the neck, place a blanket under his/her shoulders, but not under the head (it should function like a thin *Sarvāngāsana* platform).

✔ **Student:** As the helper pulls the belt, breathe slowly and deeply to open your chest. Observe how much the upper parts of the lungs participate in the breathing.

Setu Bandha Sarvāngāsana

Variation 4
Learning to arch back from Sarvāngāsana: Using the wall

Effects

For many people arching back to Setu Bandha from Sarvāngāsana is frightening, since it requires dropping back to the invisible. The vicinity of the wall helps to overcome this fear. It also limits the extent of the arching. The distance from the wall can be increased as one becomes familiar and gains confidence with the required actions.

If the chest region is not sufficiently elastic the final pose will exert too much pressure on the wrists. This may be painful. Pushing the wall teaches one to use the legs in order to lift and open the chest. This reduces the pressure on the wrists, because the feet are higher and the push against the wall lifts the chest.

Props

5-6 blankets, belt, wall

This Variation is done as part of the *Sarvāngāsana* cycle. If you do not know how to prepare a *Sarvāngāsana* platform see Variation 1 of *Sālamba Sarvāngāsana* on page 62.

➤ To find the position of the platform relative to the wall, sit in *Dandāsana* on the platform with your feet against the wall ❶.

> ***Note:*** the head-side (rounded edge) of the platform should point away from the wall.

The farther the platform is from the wall, the more you will have to arch back in order to reach the wall. Start with a shorter distance and with practice, increase it, until finally you will be able to lower the feet to the floor (or to a bolster placed near the wall).

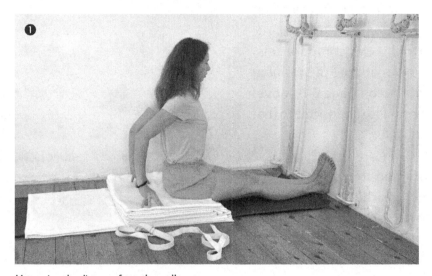

Measuring the distance from the wall

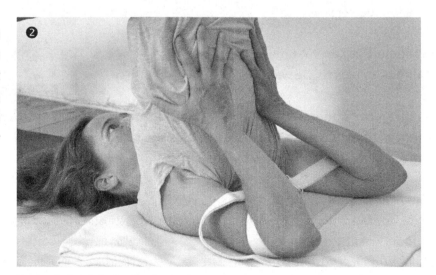

Turning the hands for *Setu Bandha Sarvāngāsana*

Setu Bandha Sarvāngāsana

Variation 4 (Cont'd)
Learning to arch back from Sarvāngāsana: Using the wall

To arch back from *Sarvāngāsana*:

→ Go up and stay in *Sarvāngāsana* for a few minutes.

> Turn the hands such that the fingers are pointing up toward the buttocks ❷. (compare this with ❹ in Variation 1 of *Sālamba Sarvāngāsana* on page 64). Move the palms as close as possible to the shoulder blades.

> Arch back and move the left leg down until it reaches the wall. Stretch the right leg vertically up ❸. This is *Eka Pāda Setu Bandha Sarvāngāsana* (LOY Pl. 260).

> Now lower the right leg to the wall and lift the left leg vertically up.

> You can repeat this several times. Finally bring both legs to the wall.

> Push the feet against the wall and move the top chest closer to the chin ❹.

> Stay in *Setu Bandha Sarvāngāsana* for 1 to 3 minutes, and then go back to *Sālamba Sarvāngāsana*; continue with *Halāsana*, *Karnapidāsana* and other variations of the *Sarvāngāsana* cycle.

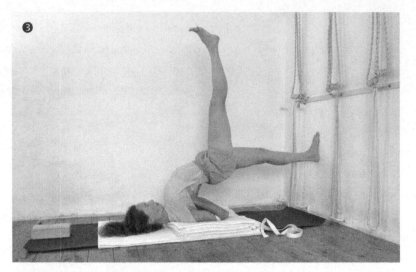

❸

Eka Pāda Setu Bandha Sarvāngāsana – one leg against wall

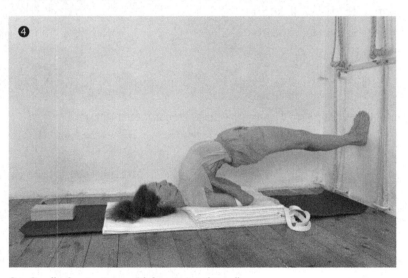

❹

Setu Bandha Sarvāngāsana with feet against the wall

T i p s
✔ When pushing the wall with the feet, do not allow the shoulders to slide off of the platform; only move the chest closer to the head. If the shoulders slip, place a sticky-piece under them.

✔ Push the feet against the wall to move the chest until the chin touches the notch between the collar bones (this is *Jālandhara Bandha*).

✔ To ease the pose you may start by spreading the legs slightly, and gradually join them.

Setu Bandha Sarvāngāsana

Variation 5
Activating the legs and arms: Pulling a belt

Effects
The belt helps to activate the legs and the arms. Pulling the belt moves the shoulders toward the legs and activates the muscles of the back and to lift the chest.

Props
1-2 belts, block (optional)

In this active Variation, the hands are holding a belt looped around the feet.

➡️ Loop a belt and place it on the mat. Sit next to it and place the feet inside the loop.

› Take the far strip of the belt and move it in between the lower legs.

› Now lie down on the mat. Bend the knees and catch the belt at a distance of approximately 40 cm (1 foot) from the feet.

› Hold the belt firmly and stretch the legs to lift the pelvis as high as possible.

› Lift the chest by pushing the legs against the belt.

› Move the shoulders toward the heels and roll the outer shoulders down to press the floor. Move the sternum up and toward the face.

› Stay in the pose breathing deeply and smoothly.

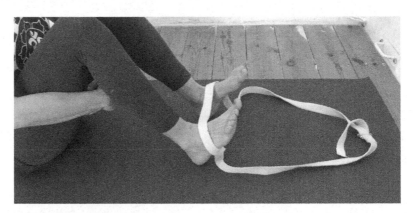

Placing the belt on the feet

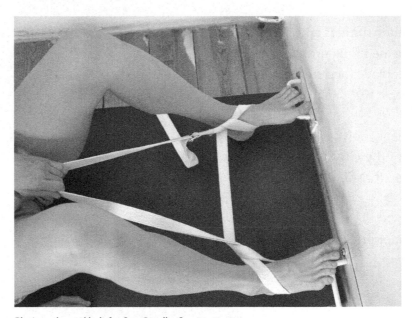

Placing a looped belt for *Setu Bandha Sarvāngāsana*

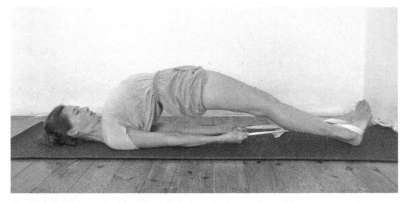

Setu Bandha Sarvāngāsana pulling a belt

Variation 5 (Cont'd)
Activating the legs and arms:
Pulling a belt

You can do this Variation with two belts; tighten one on the right foot, and the other on the left foot:

→ Tighten each belt around both feet such that the open edge of each belt extends sideways ❶.

❯ Lie down, bend the knees and catch the belts ❷.

❯ Then straighten the legs and lift the pelvis. Move the shoulders back; lift the shoulder blades and sternum to open the chest ❸.

You can use the belts to improve the opening of the chest also in the supported version of *Setu Bandha Sarvāngāsana* ❹.

With a block support, you can do also *Viparīta Karaṇi* ❺.

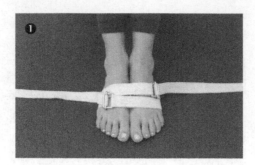

Placing a belt on each foot

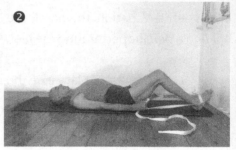

Preparing for active *Setu Bandha Sarvāngāsana*

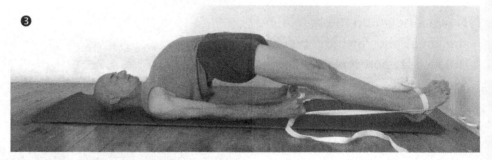

Setu Bandha Sarvāngāsana pulling two belts

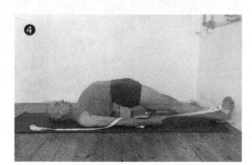

With block support

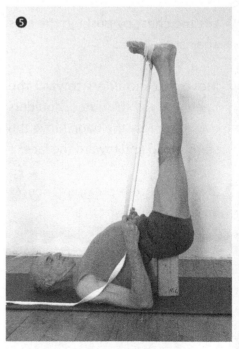

Viparīta Karaṇi on block, pulling belts

Restorative
Setu Bandha Sarvāngāsana

The following Variations are very relaxing; they open the chest without activating the muscles; hence, they can be used to lower the blood pressure and to quiet the mind. Guruji Iyengar writes in the *Effects* for this pose in LOY: "*A healthy and flexible spine indicates a healthy nervous system. If the nerves are healthy a man is sound in mind and body.*"

These Variations are very suitable for women during menses and can be practiced as a replacement for *Sarvāngāsana*. During menstruation, it is recommended to raise the feet to the level of the pelvis and to ensure that the abdomen is absolutely soft.

Setu Bandha Sarvāngāsana

Variation 6
Pelvis on foam blocks, back supported

Effects
This is a very relaxing way to do Setu Bandha Sarvāngāsana. Both the pelvis and the back are supported by a wide and soft support, which makes the pose very soothing.

Props
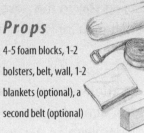
4-5 foam blocks, 1-2 bolsters, belt, wall, 1-2 blankets (optional), a second belt (optional)

In this restorative Variation the pelvis rests on a stack of 4 foam blocks. Any similar support can be used (A *Viparīta Karaṇi* box is especially designed for it, so, if you have one, use it).

→ Place a pile of 4-5 foam blocks at an appropriate distance from the wall. If the pile is unstable, wrap a belt around the blocks and tighten it to prevent slippage (not shown).

> Lean a bolster on the head side of the foam blocks.

> Place another bolster widthwise next to the wall for heels support (this is optional; you can rest the heels on the floor).

> Sit on the foam blocks and tighten a belt around your upper thighs.

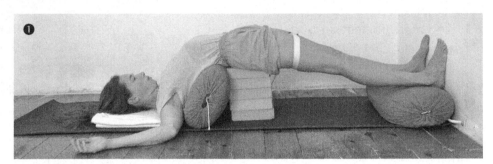
Setu Bandha Sarvāngāsana with foam blocks & bolsters

> Arch the back on the bolster and rest the shoulders, the neck and the back of the head on the floor. If the shoulders do not reach the floor, fill the gap with one or two folded blankets as shown in ❶.

> Extend the legs and place the feet on the bolster and against the wall.

> Roll the shoulders back (toward the wall), and move the outer shoulders down to the floor ❶.

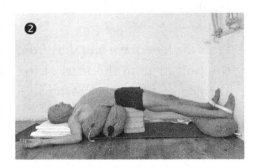
Using two bolsters to support the chest

Tips
✓ Tall people can use an extra bolster ❷, or lean a few folded blankets against the first bolster. Photo ❷ also shows strapping the feet instead of the thighs.

Effects

The bolster supports the entire back and hence this is a very relaxing Variation. The upper back is arched and breathing is automatically directed to the top chest. Beginners can learn the basics of Prāṇāyāma in this variation.

Props

bolster, block, belt, wall, blanket (optional)

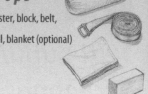

This is a milder version of the previous variation; it requires fewer props and is suitable for beginners and for people with limited movement in the upper back. It is also suitable for a longer and relaxed stay in the pose. It is a good preparation for *Prāṇāyāma*.

→ Spread the mat perpendicular to the wall. Place the bolster on top of a folded blanket centered lengthwise on the mat.

❯ Place a block (for feet support) next to the wall.

❯ Lie with your back and shoulders on the bolster and tighten a belt around your upper thighs.

❯ Bend the legs and place the feet on the floor.

❯ Press the feet down and slide from the bolster until the tops of the shoulders and the back of the neck and head are on the floor ❶.

❯ Now straighten the legs and place the feet on the block and against the wall ❷.

❯ Roll the shoulders back and open the chest. Stay in the pose, breathing softly and smoothly.

❯ Another option is to spread the legs ❸.

❯ A rolled blanket or towel can be placed to support the back of the neck – this allows for a better relaxation of the neck and throat ❸.

> *Note:* Place the bolster as far as possible from the wall, provided that the shoulders reach the floor. If the bolster is too close to the wall, the chest will not be lifted and opened sufficiently.

❯ If you find the bolster is not in place, lift your body supporting it on the feet and elbows and move the bolster to the correct position ❹.

Tips

✔ Enter the pose by sliding to the head side. This creates natural arching of the upper back.

✔ After reaching the floor, release the skin of the front and outer shoulders down to the floor. It is essential that the shoulders are well rested, and the face is directed toward the chest.

✔ If the shoulders do not reach the floor after adjusting the bolster's position, place a folded blanket under the shoulders.

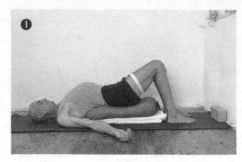

Entering *Setu Bandha Sarvāngāsana* on bolster – knees bent

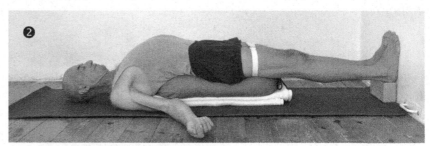

Setu Bandha Sarvāngāsana on a spine-wise bolster

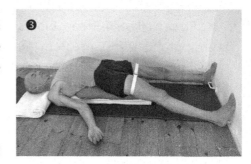

Setu Bandha Sarvāngāsana spreading the legs

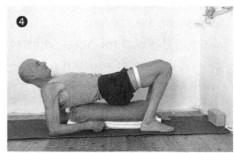

Adjusting the bolster position in *Setu Bandha Sarvāngāsana*

Setu Bandha Sarvāngāsana

Variation 8
Soft Support:
Using a support of several bolsters

Effects
This is an extremely enjoyable Variation! The soft and wide support enables the back muscle to soften and widen. It is useful when a deep relaxation is needed.

Props
6 bolsters or 4 bolsters and 4 foam blocks, belt, 2-3 blankets

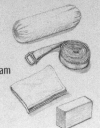

→ Prepare 3 pairs of bolsters; each pair is formed by a bolster on top of another. Place the bolsters widthwise (parallel to the wall).

❯ Adjust the bolsters such that first pair supports the back; the second supports the pelvis and the third pair supports the feet.

> *Note:* The third pair, which supports the feet, may be replaced by another type of support, e.g. foam blocks.

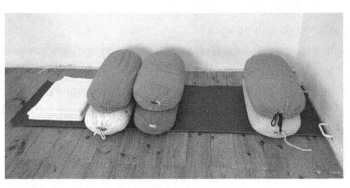

Six bolster arrangement for wide support

❯ If needed, prepare 1 to 3 folded blankets next to the first pair of bolsters, for shoulders and head support.

❯ Sit on the second (middle) pair of bolsters.

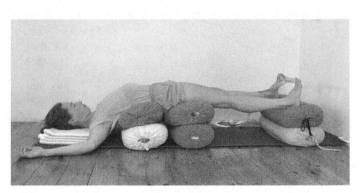

Setu Bandha Sarvāngāsana on wide support

❯ With knees bent and feet on the floor, slide back until the shoulders are resting on the floor (or on the folded blankets).

❯ Stretch the legs and rest the feet on the third pair of bolsters. Loop a belt around the big toes to keep the big toes slightly tilted towards each other. Spread the heels sideways.

❯ Stay in the pose, breathing softly and smoothly.

Pīncha Mayūrāsana

About Pīncha Mayūrāsana

Pīncha Mayūrāsana - the Peacock's Feather pose (LOY Pl. 357) - is more advanced and challenging than Sirsāsana. It requires more strength and movement in the shoulders, as well as a balancing ability. It develops balance, confidence and lightness (as its name implies). Although more challenging than Sirsāsana, it can serve as a preparation for it. In fact, it is only after achieving some control in Pīncha Mayūrāsana that one should attempt staying 10 minutes or more in Sirsāsana. This is because both poses require pushing the forearms down in order to lift the shoulders and activate the upper arms and the back muscles, which in turn keeps the shoulder blades in and opens the chest. These actions transfer the body's weight to the arm bones. Learning to do it in Pīncha Mayūrāsana, in which the head does not touch the floor, will help you protect the neck in Sirsāsana.

Pīncha Mayurāsana

Variation 1
Preparations for the pose

Effects

These preparations create flexibility in the shoulder girdle and teach one to use the forearms in Pīncha Mayurāsana.

Props

wall, block, belt

(optional)

Preparation I: Forearms on wall

Three positions of the hands are shown in this preparation (these are equivalent to the possible hands positions when doing the pose on the floor).

→ Stand facing the wall, about 60 cm (2 feet) away from it.

❯ Place a block between the palms and press them against it. Lean forward to place the forearms on the wall, elbows higher than shoulder level and shoulder-width apart.

> *Note:* The arms should be parallel to each other. If the elbows slip away from each other, place a shoulder-width belt around the elbows.

❯ Push against the wall and move the chest away from the wall to extend the armpits.

❯ Connect the upper arms with the shoulder blades and move the shoulder blades inward.

❯ Make the upper back concave and move the forehead toward the wall. Keep the head in between the upper arms.

❯ After staying in the pose for a minute or so, move the head slightly away from the wall and turn the palms such that the backs of the hands are placed on the wall. Hold the block by pressing the outer palms (little finger side) against it.

❯ Press the outer elbows to the wall. Try to touch the wall with the nails of the thumbs. Extend the inner arms from the inner elbows to the armpits.

❯ Connect the humerus bones to the shoulders and make the back concave to move the forehead toward the wall.

❯ Now keeping the outer elbows pressing against the wall, roll the hands and place the palms against the wall. Press the inner hands (thumb sides) against the block.

❯ Again move the trunk away from the wall and make the back concave.

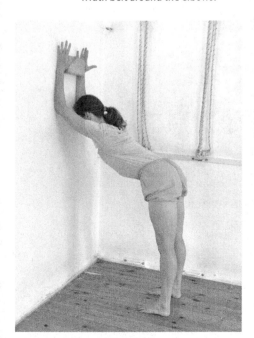

Pīncha Mayurāsana preparation 1
– palms against the blocks

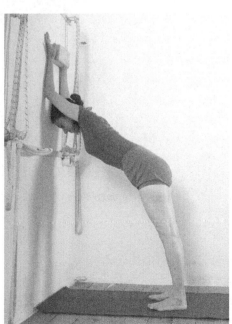

Pīncha Mayurāsana preparation 1
– backs of hands against wall

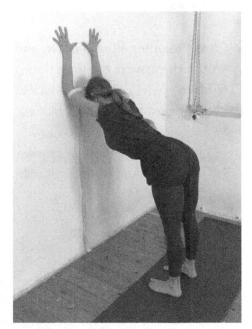

Pīncha Mayurāsana preparation 1
– palms against wall

Pīncha Mayurāsana

Variation 1 (Cont'd)
Preparations for the pose

Preparation II: Elbows on floor, forearms against wall

→ Kneel next to the wall. Place a block in between the outer hands (little finger side) and press against it.

❯ Place the elbows on the floor and press them against the wall. Move the forearms evenly toward the wall until the backs of the hands and the block touch the wall.

❯ Now straighten the knees and step forward. Move the shoulder blades away from the wall and make the back concave.

❯ Keeping the back concave, lift the pelvis and step as close as possible to the wall.

❯ Press the outer elbows down and lift the chest; work the front thighs to lift the pelvis. Allow the block to press against the shoulder blades.

> *Note:* If the elbows slip and widen, use a belt to keep them right under the shoulders.

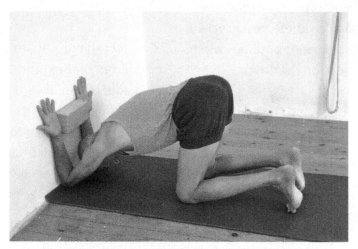

Pīncha Mayurāsana preparation 2 – placing the elbows in the corner

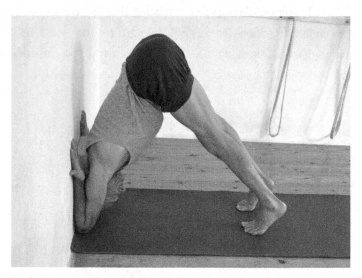

Pīncha Mayurāsana preparation 2 – (elbows in the corner)

Preparation III: *Adho Mukha Śvānāsana* on the forearms

This preparation is called *Ardha Pīncha Mayurāsana* (see: *Yoga in Action, Intermediate Course-I* P. 62).

→ Put a shoulder-width belt just above the elbows.

> Place the forearms and hands on the floor and hold a block between the hands.

T i p s

✔ Photo ❶ shows placing the back of the hands down - this helps to roll the biceps out and to press the outer elbows down. There are other options to position the hands against the block, e.g.: palms on the floor ❷, outer hands on the floor (Sirsāsana-hands). Try these options and observe the differences.

> Raise the knees up, lift the heels and anchor the toes.

> Push the forearms and hands down to move the rest of the body back and up. Move the front thighs back to extend the spine backward.

> Walk in with the feet while moving the shoulder blades in to make the back as concave as possible ❶.

> Then keeping the buttocks lifted, lower the heels down ❷.

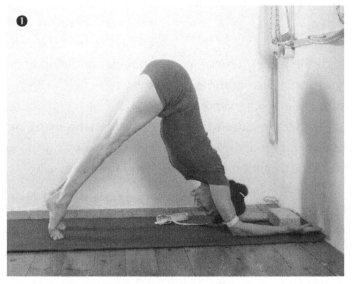

Pīncha Mayurāsana preparation 3 – back of hands on floor

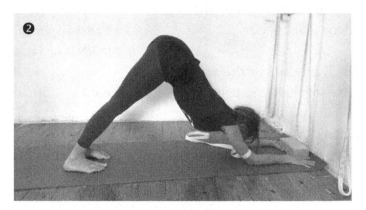

Pīncha Mayurāsana preparation 3 – palms on floor, heels down

Pīncha Mayūrāsana

Variation 2
Supporting the base:
Using block and belt

Effects

A belt for the elbows and a block between the palms stabilize the forearms and elbows and help to ground them to the floor.

Props

block or two, belt, wall

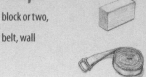

Continuing from Preparation III above, a belt and a block are used to stabilize the elbows, forearms and hands. The support of the wall helps to balance in the pose.

The stability of the base is crucial in *Pīncha Mayūrāsana*. The common tendency is for the elbows to spread wider and for the hands to slide inward. This weakens the support of the entire pose and causes the shoulders to sink.

As shown above, there are several ways to place the hands. In the standard approach, which is shown first, the palms are facing down (in prone position), pressing against the floor (like in the final pose) and the block is used to create space between the thumbs and the index fingers.

→ Place a block near the wall and kneel next to it. Place a belt just above the elbows and tighten it to keep the elbows at the width of your shoulders.

> *Note:* If your shoulders are wider than the block, use two blocks as shown in **❶**.

> Place the forearms on the floor, palms down, on either side of the block.

> Use the block to spread well the thumbs from the index fingers.

> Make sure that the forearms are parallel to each other at shoulder width.

> Press the forearms down and the elbows against the belt. Move the shoulder girdle up and away from the wall.

> Straighten the knees, step forward, but keep moving the upper back away from the wall.

> Bend one leg and use it to push and to jump up. Swing the other leg up to the wall and then lift the pushing leg to join it. Lean both heels on the wall.

> *Note:* When jumping up, use one leg to hop, keeping the other leg straight to use it as a lever.

> Push the entire forearms down, stretch the legs up and slide the heels up the wall **❷**.

> Stay in the pose from 30 to 60 seconds. Then go down, leg by leg and rest in *Adho Mukha Vīrāsana* or in *Uttānāsana* with legs joined.

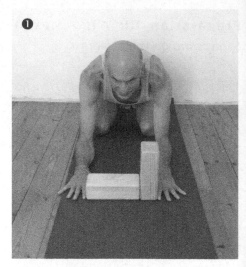

Pīncha Mayūrāsana using 2 blocks

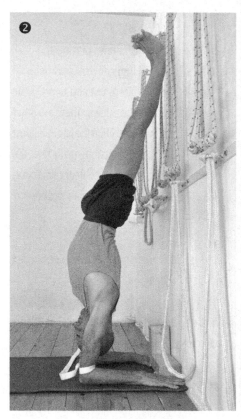

Pīncha Mayūrāsana using a belt and blocks

Once you are confident in the pose, learn to balance without the wall:

→ Move one leg away from the wall and stretch it up.

❯ Then repeat with the other leg.

❯ Finally move both legs, one by one, away from the wall and balance ❸. Keep stretching up and avoid dropping the shoulders or projecting the lower ribs forward.

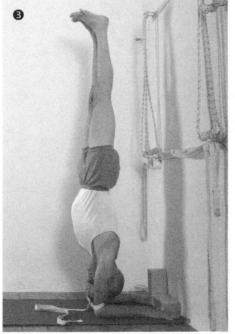

Balancing in *Pīncha Mayurāsana*

Tips

✔ Connect the upper arms to the shoulder blades and the shoulder blades to the spine. Use the legs to stretch the spine upward.

✔ Move the shoulder blades and tailbone away from the wall while moving the floating ribs, false ribs and lumbar spine toward the wall.

✔ When using the wall let the head hang loose while looking forward in parallel to the floor. Search for the vertical alignment between the crown of the head, the center of the chest, the perineum and the meeting point of the ankles.

✔ When doing the pose away from the wall, it is easier to balance with the eyes looking at the floor. Extend the cervical spine and arch the neck to look down. To keep your balance, push the shoulder blades in and maintain the vertical alignment between the center of the chest, the perineum and the ankles.

There are more ways to use the block to get different effects. Here are three such options:

I. **Palms against the block – (hands like *Sirsāsana*)**

Effects: *Pressing the palms against the block and pushing the sides of the forearms (ulna bones) against the floor strengthens the arms and prepares for Sirsāsana.*

→ Place a block in between the palms. Press the outer palms down to the floor and the palms against the block ❶.

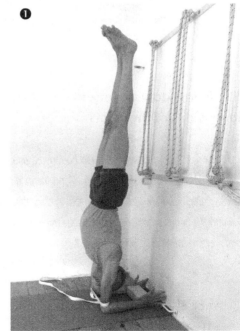

Pīncha Mayurāsana – palms against block

Variation 2 (Cont'd)
Supporting the base:
Using block and belt

II. Palms facing up

Effects: *Turning the hands helps to roll the biceps out and to press down the outer sides of the elbows down. These are important actions in Pīncha Mayurāsana*

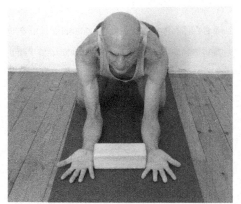

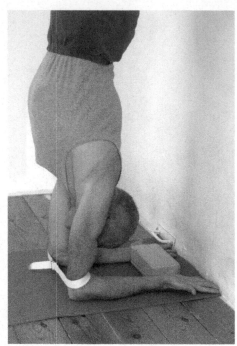

Turning the hands

Palms facing up

III. Palms down; block in between inner sides of the wrists

Effects: *To get stability in Pīncha Mayurāsana one should press both the outer elbows and the inner sides of the wrists down. This variation teaches this. Turning the hands slightly out activates the upper arms and prevents the elbows from sliding out.*

⟶ Place a block in between the inner sides (thumb sides) of the wrists.

❯ Press the inner wrists and thumbs against the block and widen the fingers apart.

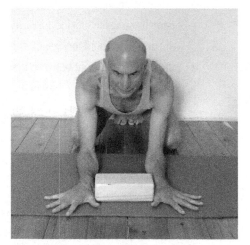

Palms down and turned out

❯ If the elbows tend to slip and widen apart, place on them a shoulder-width belt.

❯ Go up to the pose.

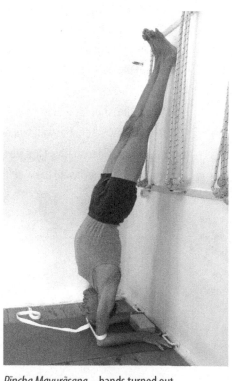

Pīncha Mayurāsana – hands turned out

Pincha Mayurāsana

Variation 3
Moving the tailbone in:
Feet against wall

Effects
Pushing the wall enables you to lift the buttocks and to move the tailbone in.

Props
block or two, belt, wall

→ Arrange the props (blocks and belt) as in the previous Variation, but place the block(s) about 30 cm (1 foot) away from the wall.

〉 Go up to the pose and place the feet against the wall with bent knees. ❶.

〉 Push the wall to lift the buttocks and move the tailbone in ❷.

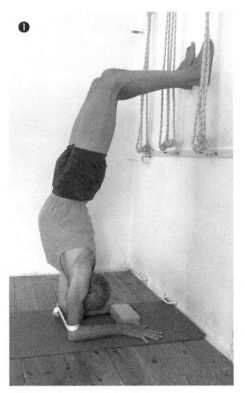

Feet against wall

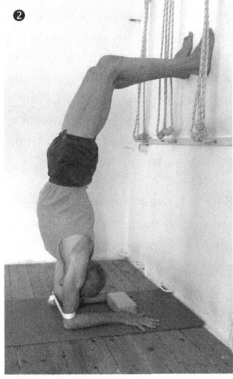

Pushing the tailbone in

Variation 4
Moving weight to the palms:
Supporting the elbows

Effects

The support for the elbows shifts weight to the palms, thus creating a better base for the pose.

Props

folded sticky mat, block, belt, wall

One of the challenges of the pose is to shift weight from the elbows to the roots of the palms, such that the load of the body is distributed across the entire length of the forearms. Elevating the elbow on a support shifts weight to the palms and makes the foundation of the pose stronger.

➡️ Take a 4-folded sticky mat and fold it by three. Place the resulting sticky strip across the mat at the appropriate distance from the wall (your forearms' length).

❯ Use the belt and block as in the previous Variation.

❯ Place the elbows on the sticky strip and go up to *Pīncha Mayurāsana*, as explained above.

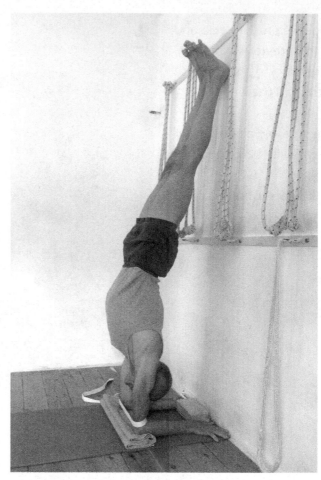

Pīncha Mayurāsana using a belt, block and folded mat for elbows

Tips

✔ Press the outer elbows and the inner wrists down to the floor.

Pīncha Mayūrāsana

Variation 5
Stabilizing the palms:
Using a weight

Effects

The weight grounds the hands to the floor; this makes the pose more stable and enables a longer stay with less effort. Turning the hands up helps to roll the biceps out.

Props

metal weight, belt, wall (optional)

→ Place a weight of 10 to 20 kg (20 to 45 lbs.) on the mat. Insert the forearms under the weight with the palms facing up at shoulder width ❶.

❯ Go up to the pose ❷.

Notes:

1. You can also do this Variation with the palms facing down, resembling the final pose.

2. If available, ask a helper to put the weight on your palms after placing the arms on the floor.

A helper can produce a similar effect by stepping on the practitioner's hands ❸. This is done with the student's palms facing down.

Instructions for the helper:

→ After the practitioner places her/his forearms on the floor, step carefully on the inner (thumb) side of the hands.

❯ Then help her/him to come up to the pose.

❯ To provide further help, gently catch the false ribs of the practitioner and move them up and back.

❶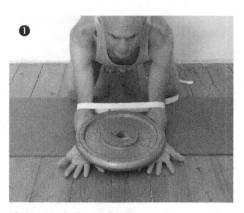

Placing weight for Pīncha Mayūrāsana

❷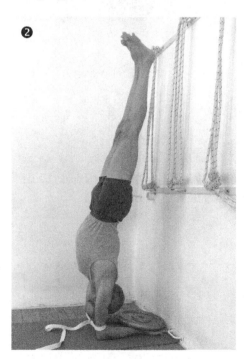

Pīncha Mayūrāsana with weight on palms

❸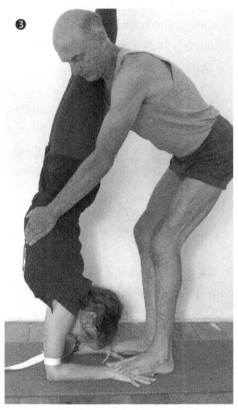

Help in Pīncha Mayūrāsana

Variation 6
Moving the shoulder blades in: Using a chair

Effects

The chair keeps the shoulder blades lifted and tucked in; this allows lifting the rib cage without dropping the upper arms and shoulders. It also helps to sense the alignment of the shoulder blades.

Props

wall, chair. Optional: belt, block

This Variation is similar to Variation 10 of *Sirsāsana* (page 28); however here there is no need to elevate the base of the pose, since in *Pīncha Mayūrāsana* the shoulder blades band is usually at the level of the seat.

→ Place the chair with its back against the wall. Optionally you can place a sticky mat on the seat for cushioning.

> **Note:** If there is a space between the backrest and the wall, the chair may tilt; to prevent this, fill the gap by a foam block or any other material.

> Optionally you can use a belt for the elbows and a block for the hands.

> Place the forearms under the chair and go up to the pose.

> **Tips**
> ✓ If the distance from the chair is not correct, go down and adjust, until the edge of the seat supports your shoulder blades without pushing you too far forward.

> Place the heels on the wall, stretch the legs and lift the sternum and the front ribs.

> Lift the buttocks and tighten them in.

> You can try to balance by moving one leg at a time away from the wall.

> Stretch the legs vertically up.

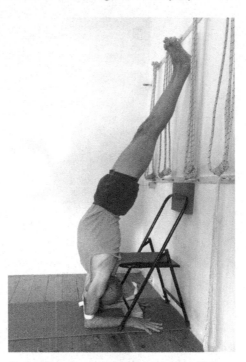

Pīncha Mayūrāsana with chair for shoulder blades – heels on wall

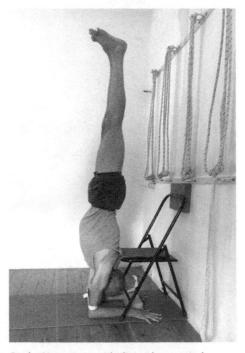

Pīncha Mayūrāsana with chair – legs vertical

Adho Mukha Vṛkṣāsana

"They speak of the imperishable Aśvatthām (peepal tree) as having its root above and branches below. Its leaves are the Vedas and who knows this is the knower of the Vedas."

This verse from the *Bhagavad-Gītā* (XV.I) describes an inverted tree as a symbol of the world as a living organism, united with the Supreme. This image resembles *Adho Mukha Vṛkṣāsana* – the "downward facing tree pose" – with the hands being the branches and the feet the roots.

Adho Mukha Vṛkṣāsana, the full-arms balance (LOY Pl. 359) is an energizing and dynamic inverted pose, which is often used for warming-up in the beginning of a practice session, as it activates the entire body and the breath. Even beginners, who cannot do *Sirsāsana*, can practice this pose since it is easier to move the shoulders when the arms are straight, and there is no risk of injuring the neck. I show a few variations for strengthening the arms and building confidence in the pose.

Taking load on the bones of the arms is very beneficial for their health. In our daily life, we need to use the legs (even if it is only to walk from the car to the office…), but we rarely put load on the arms. Yoga offers many hand balancing poses. We have already seen one - *Pīncha Mayurāsana*. *Adho Mukha Vṛkṣāsana* is another example of those hand balancing poses, which are nick-named 'bird poses.'

Learning *Adho Mukha Vṛkṣāsana*

In learning this pose one may face physical as well as psychological difficulties. The next two Variations help to overcome those.

Adho Mukha Vṛkṣāsana

Variation 1
*Strengthening the arms:
Climbing on the wall*

Effects

This Variation strengthens the arms and builds confidence; it demonstrates (for those who are not sure) that the arms are strong enough to carry the body weight.

Props

wall

Many students are not sure whether they can bear their body weight on the arms. Here is a safe way to prove it for yourself.

> Stand with your back to the wall, about 1 meter (3 feet) away from it. Bend forward to place the palms on the floor.

> Place the palms equidistant from the wall, shoulder width apart, middle fingers pointing forward, parallel to each other. Spread the fingers well to broaden the palms.

> Now climb the legs up the wall and stretch the body up.

> Press the palms against the floor to lift the torso. Tighten the elbows to keep them straight.

> Stay for 40-45 sec. with fluent breathing. Then come down. Repeat several times.

> ✔ **Tips** To stabilize the arms, suck the biceps and the triceps to the humerus bones (of the upper arms) and keep the elbows strong and straight.

Once you are confident, decrease the distance from the wall:

> To measure the distance from the wall: sit in *Daṇḍāsana* with feet against the wall, and mark the position of your buttocks.

> Turn and place the palms at the marked position on the floor; then climb with your feet on the wall as before.

> After stretching the arms and stabilizing the shoulder blades, start stepping down the wall with straight legs. Your goal is to make a 90° angle at the pelvis, with the legs parallel to the floor and the upper body vertical.

> Push the palms against the floor, tighten and lift the front thighs and extend the upper body.

> Extend the armpits. Move the shoulder blades in to make the upper back concave.

> Stay for 40-45 sec. with fluent breathing. Then come down. Repeat 2-3 times.

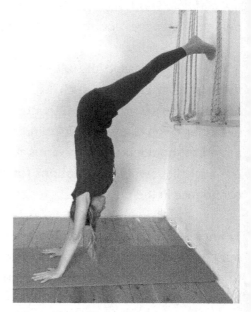

Adho Mukha Vṛkṣāsana – climbing on wall

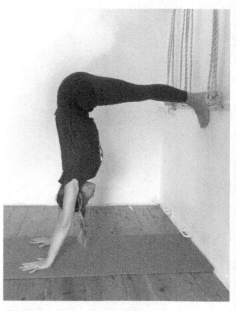

Climbing on the wall - legs at 90°

Adho Mukha Vṛkṣāsana

Variation 2
Overcoming fear:
Bolster against the wall

Effects

The soft bolster being more 'friendly' than the hard wall, helps to overcome the fear of hitting the wall when jumping up into the pose. Once up, the contact of the head with the bolster stabilizes the pose.

Props

wall, bolster

Some students, although able to carry themselves on the arms, are reluctant to jump up with the back to the wall. They are afraid of losing control and banging their head into the wall. Magically, a bolster placed against the wall helps to overcome this fear.

➡️ Place a bolster vertically against on the wall.

❯ Place the palms on either side of the bolster, equidistant from the wall and the bolster. Spread the fingers well to broaden the palms ❶.

❯ Now bend one leg and use it to jump up. Keep the other leg straight and use it to swing the body into the pose ❷.

❯ Once you are up: join the legs, push the palms down against the floor, stretch up the entire body and slide the heels up the wall.

❯ Lift the buttock bones toward the heels and move the tailbone in.

❯ Move the head forward to lengthen the back of the neck and look up as if you want to see your navel. Move the shoulder blades in and tighten them toward the back ribs. At the same time do not project the lower ribs forward, but keep them close to the wall ❸.

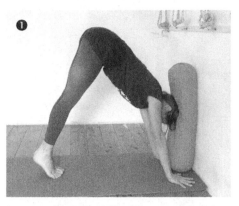

❶ Preparing for *Adho Mukha Vṛkṣāsana* with bolster leaning on the wall

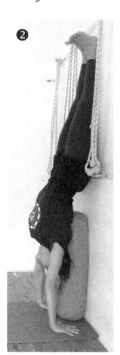 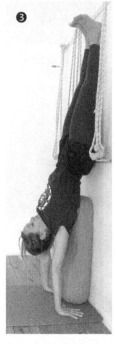

❷ Coming up with bolster support

❸ *Adho Mukha Vṛkṣāsana* – looking up to move the shoulder blades in

Tips

✔ Looking up lengthens the back of the neck and helps to move the shoulder blades in.

✔ Suck the deltoid muscles (of the shoulders) to the armpits, lift them to the shoulders and open and extend the armpits.

❯ Then release the head and let it hang. Look forward; relax the face and breathe smoothly.

❯ Stay 30-45 sec. then come down one leg at a time and recover in *Uttānāsana* with spread legs.

Tips

✔ Notice which leg you use for jumping up into the pose. Then try to jump with the other leg. Practice the pose an even number of times and change the leg each time.

✔ Once you master jumping into the pose with one leg try to jump with both legs concurrently. When doing so, concentrate on lifting the entire pelvic girdle rather than bringing your feet to the wall.

Adho Mukha Vṛkṣāsana

Variation 3
Help in lifting the legs:
Using chair to go up

Effects
People who find it hard to jump up to the pose can place the feet on the chair and use it as a springboard.

Props
chair, wall

→ Place a chair at about 1 meter (3 feet) away from the wall.

> Place the palms at shoulder width, next to the wall.

> Lift the legs to place the feet on the chair.

> Lift one leg up and stretch it up.

> Bend the other leg and use it to jump up until the heels are supported by the wall.

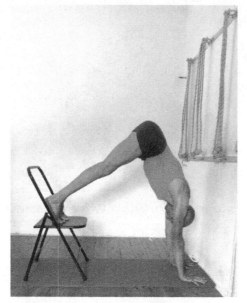

Using a chair to go up to *Adho Mukha Vṛkṣāsana*

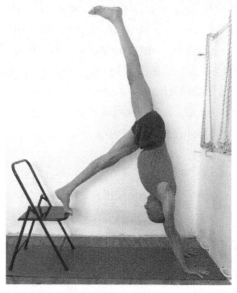

Lifting a leg from the chair

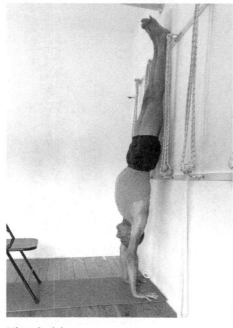

Lifting both legs

> ⚠ **CAUTIONS**
>
> When coming down make sure not to hit the chair with your legs.

Adho Mukha Vṛkṣāsana

Variation 4
Stabilizing the arms: Belt on elbows

Effects

The belt keeps the elbows straight. It helps to align the upper arms with the forearms and to keep the arms parallel and vertical. It is also reassuring to those who are scared that their elbows will buckle after some time in the pose, as they work to build the strength and stamina in the pose. The pose becomes less effortful since the body weight is borne by the bones of the arms.

Props

wall, belt

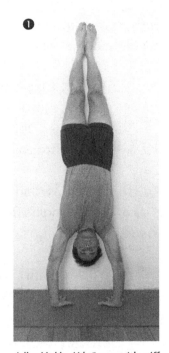

❶

Sage *Patañjali* described the quality of an *āsana* in *Sutras* 46 & 47 of *Sādhanā Pāda* very concisely and precisely as: *sthira sukham āsanam* and *prayatna shaithilya ananta samapattibhyam*.

The English translation given by Guruji Iyengar is:

> *Āsana is perfect firmness of body, steadiness of intelligence and benevolence of spirit*

> *Perfection in āsana is achieved when the effort to perform it becomes effortless and the infinite being within is reached*

One of the principles of alignment in Iyengar Yoga is that the body weight should be borne by the bones. The muscles are used to move the bones to their proper position and to stabilize the joints. The bones are considered *Earth Element* – they are solid and can provide *Sthirata* (firmness and steadiness); the muscles cannot provide stability, steadfastness and firmness for a long time. Carrying the weight on the bones reduces the muscular effort in the pose and enables one to experience *prayatna shaithilya* – the joy of 'effortless effort'.

Adho Mukha Vṛkṣāsana with stiff elbows

❷

In this Variation, the belt on the elbows helps to bring the bones of the arms to the correct vertical alignment. It is especially helpful for practitioners who have stiff elbows and shoulders and struggle to straighten the arms.

> Loop a belt to the width of your shoulders and place it on the elbows.

> Move the elbows up and toward the wall, while moving the shoulder blades away from the wall.

Note: If the belt does not allow you to release the head down, then place it on the forearms, under the elbows.

The belt helps practitioners who cannot straighten the elbows without it (as in ❶). Compare it with ❷ where the belt helps to draw the arms closer and keep them straighter.

> Go up to the pose with the heels against the wall.

> Push the palms down and extend the inner arms upward.

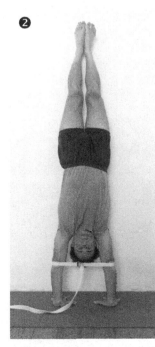

Adho Mukha Vṛkṣāsana with belt on elbows

Variation 5
*Checking the alignment:
Using a wall hook or wall corner*

Effects

The external feedback helps to judge whether the body is straight or tilted sideways.

Props

wall hook

→ Stand facing a wall equipped with hooks and place the palms equidistant from a hook.

> *Note:* Having a bottom hook in line with the top hook, as found in many Iyengar Yoga studios, helps to place the palms correctly.

❯ Go up to the pose and feel the hook ❶ or a rope hanging from it ❷ with your feet or legs.

> *Note:* After gaining some confidence in the balance you may also use an external corner to validate the vertical alignment in *Adho Mukha Vṛkṣāsana*. See Variation 6 of *Sirsāsana* (page 19) for reference.

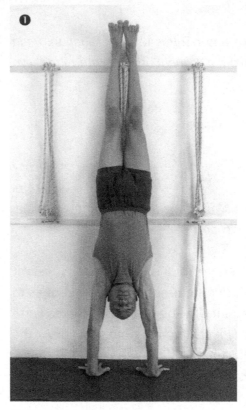

Checking the pose using hooks

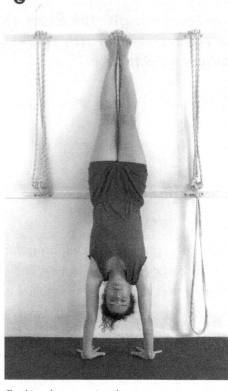

Checking the pose using the rope

Adho Mukha Vṛkṣāsana

Variation 6
Reducing wrist pressure:
Using slanting planks

Effects

Using slanting planks reduces the load on the wrist and enables doing the pose even when there is a minor wrist issue. By practicing this way, the wrist can heal, until the pose can be practiced in the usual way.

Props

wall, 1-2 slanting planks

The wrist is a vulnerable joint and many people suffer from wrist pain. In this Variation, a slanting plank is used to support the bases of the palms; this shifts weight to the finger mounds and creates more space in the wrists.

Two options are offered here:

a. Doing the pose with the palms forward (as done normally) in which case one plank is used ❶.

b. Turning the palms out and using two planks as in ❷.

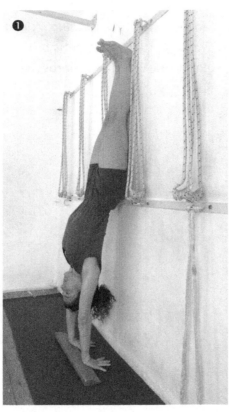

Adho Mukha Vṛkṣāsana - wrists on plank

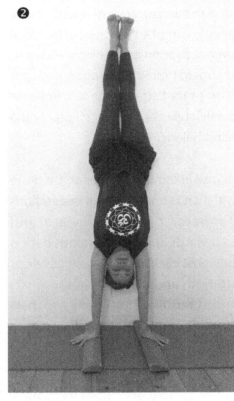

Adho Mukha Vṛkṣāsana - wrists on two planks, hands turned out

Variation 7
Different Hand Orientations: Using blocks

Turning the hands in various directions activates the wrists, elbows and shoulders in different ways. The blocks provide a firm base that activates the arms and strengthens their bones.

2 blocks, wall

In our computerized world, many people complain about wrist pain due over-activation and tension related to keyboard typing. Yoga offers plenty of *āsana-s* that strengthen and improve the flexibility of the wrists; notably, the hand balancing poses.

Adho Mukha Vṛkṣāsana can be done with hands turned in four orientations (forward, outward, inward and backward). Turning the hands back is the most challenging one. It develops strength and flexibility in the wrists and is required for *āsana-s* such as *Mayurāsana* (LOY Pl. 354) and *Setu Bandha Sarvāngāsana*; hence I start with a few preparations for this.

In *Prasārita Padottānāsana*, *Ūrdhva Mukha Śvānāsana* and *Adho Mukha Śvānāsana* the palms are on floor, but the load on the hands and wrists is much less than in *Adho Mukha Vṛkṣāsana*. Hence, these *āsana-s* can serve as a preparation for it.

→ Start with *Prasārita Padottānāsana* and turn the hands backward. Adjust the load on the palms as needed.

❯ Continue with *Ūrdhva Mukha Śvānāsana* with the hands turned back. You can place the hands on blocks to get more movement.

❯ Slowly move toward *Adho Mukha Śvānāsana*. Move the arms back to extend the wrists and improve their flexibility.

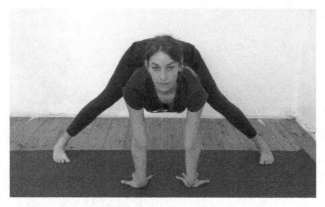

Prasārita Padottānāsana - hands turned backward

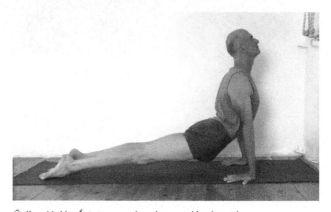

Ūrdhva Mukha Śvānāsana – hands turned backward

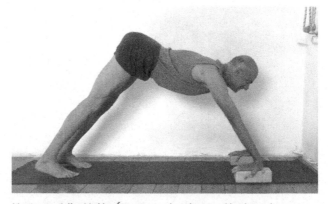

Moving to *Adho Mukha Śvānāsana* - hands turned backward

Adho Mukha Vṛksāsana variations with hands turned

The blocks help to learn these variations. It is slightly more challenging to go up to the pose with the blocks, but once you are up, the blocks provide good anchoring for the hands.

The four options are shown below:

1. Hands forward ❶

2. Hands turned outward ❷

3. Hands turned inward ❸

4. Hands turned backward ❹

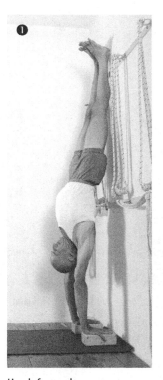

Hands forward

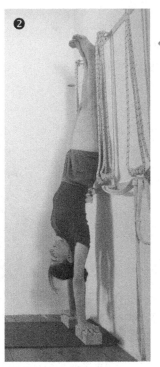

Hands turned outward

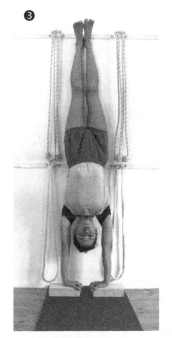

Hands turned inward

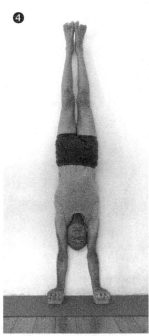

Hands turned backward

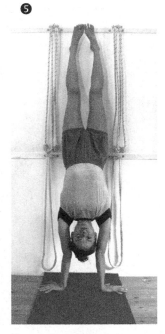

Hyperextended elbows

Tips

✓ Try these variations and study the effects of each of them on your own body. Turning the hands out, as in ❷ helps to open the shoulders and is useful when the shoulders are stiff or when it is hard to straighten the elbows. Turning the hands in, as in ❸ helps when the elbows tend to hyper-extend. People with hyperextended elbows find it hard to stabilize the elbows when the palms are facing forward or outside; since the elbows collapse in (see ❺). Turning the palms inside as in ❸ helps to control this tendency and to maintain an even length of the inner and outer arms (compare photos ❺ with ❸). Turning the hands in also helps to straighten the arms for those who are unable to straighten them due to stiffness.

Adho Mukha Vṛkṣāsana

Variation 8
Stabilizing the upper arms:
Using chairs

Effects

The chairs stabilize the upper arms and enable better access to the shoulder region. The support of the chair helps to practice the Eka Pāda variation of this pose.

Props

a chair or two, wall

→ Place two chairs with their backs against the wall. Keep a space of about 20 cm (8 inches) between the chairs for the head.

> **Note:** A single chair can be used, but you have to make sure that you do not hit the head against the seat.

> Place the palms under the chairs and go up to *Adho Mukha Vṛkṣāsana* (side view ❶; front view ❷).

> You can also try to lower one leg to *Eka Pāda Adho Mukha Vṛkṣāsana* ❸.

Effects: *Lowering one leg to Eka Pāda challenges your strength and stability and strengthens the arms and shoulders.*

> ***T i p s***
> ✓ Press the heel of the lifted leg against the wall and slide it up the wall.

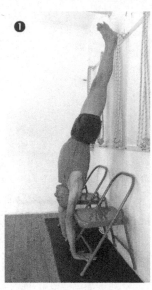

Adho Mukha Vṛkṣāsana with chairs supporting the upper arms

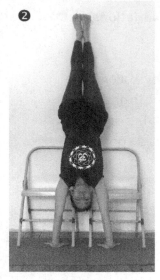

Adho Mukha Vṛkṣāsana with chairs supporting the upper arms

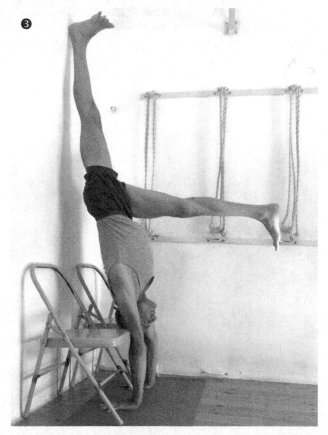

Eka Pāda Adho Mukha Vṛkṣāsana with chairs supporting the upper arms

Adho Mukha Vṛkṣāsana

Variation 9
Balance & Stability:
Learning to stand without the wall

Effects
Balancing without the wall is a great way to improve balance and control. It develops good concentration and brings about poise and lightness. It also develops the musculature of the hands, palms and fingers.

Props
wall, helper

Balancing in this pose without the wall is not common in Iyengar Yoga classes. However, personally I feel that being dependent on the wall is a drawback. The challenge of balancing on the palms in the middle of the room (or out in nature) is a great lesson and when you balance physically, there is also an accompanying mental balance and poise. The pose becomes less muscular because you balance on the bones; there is a feeling of lightness and control which does not happen when you rely on the wall.

You can learn to balance next to the wall by moving one leg at a time away from the wall and trying to balance without touching the wall. But at a certain stage you must attempt the pose without any wall nearby. If you are on your own, you will first need to learn how to fall gracefully, in case you cannot find the balance.

A good way to detach from the wall is to do the pose slightly away from the wall:

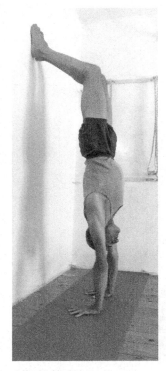 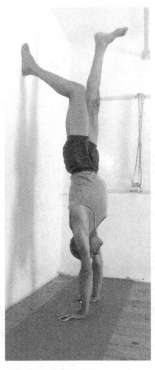 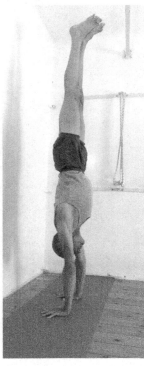

Adho Mukha Vṛkṣāsana –
learning to balance; knees bent,
feet on wall

Adho Mukha Vṛkṣāsana -
one foot on wall

Balancing

⟶ Place the palms about 50 cm (20 inches) away from the wall.

❯ As you go up to the pose, bend your knees and place the feet against the wall.

❯ First straighten one leg and stretch it vertically up.

❯ Then straighten the other leg. Stretch both legs vertically up and balance.

❯ If you lose balance, bend one leg and use the wall to restore your balance.

Tips
✓ Looking down to the floor helps to learn to balance.

Variation 9 (Cont'd)
Balance & Stability:
Learning to stand without the wall

If a helper is available, she/he can help you to learn to balance faster:

Instruction for the helper:

→ Stand close to the back of the student (when she/he is bending to get ready to jump up) **❶**.

❯ Be ready to support the student when she/he swings up and prevent her/him from falling backward.

❯ When the student comes up, support her/his heels with one hand and brace her/his front upper thighs with the other hand **❷**.

As the pose becomes somewhat stable, insert your palm (flat or fisted) in between the student's middle thighs and allow her/him to find the delicate balance on her/his own; use the other hand for extra support only when needed **❸**.

Finally, if the pose is fully stable, remove your hand, but stay there ready to help.

T i p s

✔ Spread the palms well and distribute your weight between the bases of the palms, finger mounds and fingertips.

✔ Press the tips of the fingers down; this will enlarge the area upon which you can balance (ultimately, your center of gravity must be above the palms).

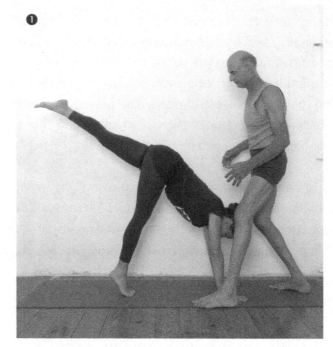

❶

Learning to balance with a helper

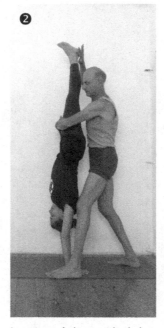

❷

Learning to balance with a helper

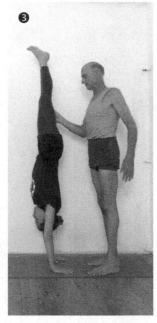

❸

Inserting one hand in between thighs

Adho Mukha Vṛksāsana

Variation 10
Restorative Adho Mukha Vṛksāsana: Supporting the head

Effects
This Variation is a combination of Sirsāsana and Adho Mukha Vṛksāsana. The support for the head makes the stay in the pose much more relaxed, and one can easily extend the stay up to 3 minutes or more.

Props
3 bolsters or 5-6 foam blocks or 2-3 wooden blocks, blankets (optional)

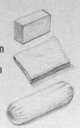

➡️ Place 2-3 bolsters on top of each other next to the wall ❶, or a pile of 6 foam blocks ❷ or three wooden blocks one on top of the other ❸.

❯ Place the palms on both sides of the support.

❯ Go up to the pose.

❶

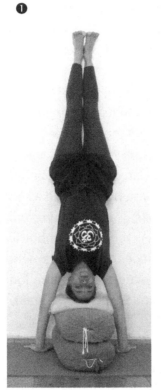

Adho Mukha Vṛksāsana - bolsters support

❷

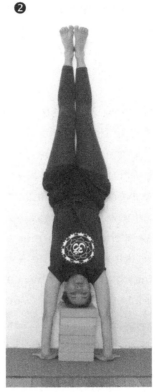

Adho Mukha Vṛksāsana - foam blocks support

❸

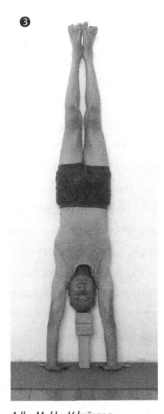

Adho Mukha Vṛksāsana - wooden blocks support

Tips

✔ Do *Ūrdhva Hastāsana* to estimate the distance from the top of the head to the wrists. The height of the support should match this distance.

✔ Do 2-3 attempts and if necessary adjust the height of the support by adding or removing blankets, until you feel that the head is supported but there is no compression in the neck.

Viparīta Karaṇi

About *Viparīta Karaṇi*

Viparīta Karaṇi is a Sanskrit term that refers to the "action of inverting" (*Viparīta* – 'inverted' or 'reversed' and *Karaṇi* – 'doing' or 'making'). Thus, it is more of a general action rather than a specific *āsana* and hence its name does not end with '*āsana*.'

Commonly, *Viparīta Karaṇi* is done in a restorative way in its '*Sarvāṅgāsana* version', where the shoulders and back of the head are on the floor, the pelvis is supported by a bolster, and the legs are resting on the wall. This is a very beneficial and relaxing restorative pose, and I explain later a way of doing it (see Variation 7 below). However, *Viparīta Karaṇi* can also be practiced as an active pose as part of the *Adho Mukha Vṛkṣāsana* cycle, *Pīncha Mayūrāsana* cycle or *Sirsāsana* cycle. In all of these, the upper back is vertical, the thoracic spine is curved and the pelvis is horizontal. These variations create movement in the shoulders and open the chest; hence they can be used as a preparation for back bends as well as for inversions like *Sirsāsana* and *Pīncha Mayūrāsana*.

Note: The active Variations of *Viparīta Karaṇi* described here are advanced. Do not attempt them if you are not confident in the inverted poses.

Viparīta Karaṇī

Variation 1
Adho Mukha Vṛkṣāsana Viparīta Karaṇī: Using the wall

Effects

Creates movement in the shoulders region and opens the chest.

Props

wall, optional:

helper, rope or belt

→ Start by placing the palms about 50 cm (1.5 foot) away from the wall and go up to *Adho Mukha Vṛkṣāsana*, heels supported by the wall.

> Move the upper arms and shoulder blades away from the wall and look up to the ceiling.

> Without disturbing the verticality of the arms, curve the thoracic spine to rest the buttocks on the wall.

> Maintain the verticality of the arms and upper back, while descending the buttocks, until the sacral band is horizontal.

> Keep moving the upper back away from the wall and stretch the legs up, along the wall. Stay from 30 seconds to a minute.

> Then go down, rest for a while and do the pose again, this time placing the palms a bit further from the wall.

Increasing the curvature with a helper

The further you are from the wall, the stronger is the curve of the back. If you find it difficult to keep the shoulders away from the wall, ask a friend to help you to stabilize the shoulder girdle.

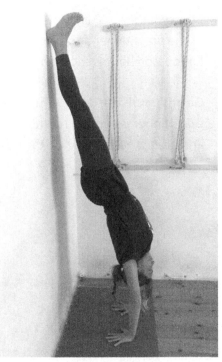

Adho Mukha Vṛkṣāsana Viparīta Karaṇī – stage 1 heels on wall

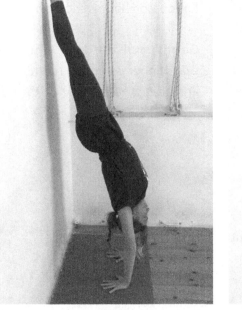

Adho Mukha Vṛkṣāsana Viparīta Karaṇī

Instructions for the helper:

> Once the practitioner is in *Adho Mukha Vṛkṣāsana* with heels against the wall, step in front of her/him and place a belt (or rope) on her/his shoulder blades.

> Gently pull the belt while the practitioner is curving her/his back and places the buttocks on the wall.

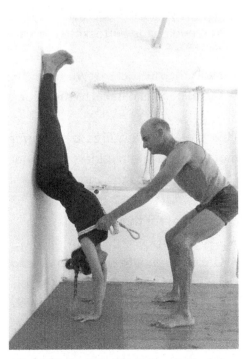

Adho Mukha Vṛkṣāsana Viparīta Karaṇī with a helper

Viparīta Karaṇi

Variation 2
Pīncha Mayurāsana Viparīta Karaṇi: Using the wall

Effects

Creates movement in the shoulders region and opens the chest.

Props

wall, helper, block, 2 belts

⟶ Place a block against the wall and a belt on the elbows as in Variation 2 of *Pīncha Mayurāsana* (on page 112).

﹥ Place the forearms on the floor about 40 cm (15 inches) away from the wall.

﹥ Go up to *Pīncha Mayurāsana* placing the heels against the wall.

﹥ Move the upper arms and shoulder blades away from the wall. Without disturbing the verticality of the arms, curve the thoracic spine to rest the buttocks on the wall.

﹥ Push the chest forward and make the upper back concave while descending the buttocks to the wall.

﹥ Slide the buttocks down until the sacral band is parallel to the floor.

This variation requires a stronger movement in the shoulders. A partner can help to create this movement.

Instructions for the helper:

﹥ Once the practitioner is in *Pīncha Mayurāsana* with her/his heels against the wall, sit in front of her/him.

﹥ Place your feet against the elbows of the practitioner and place a belt (or rope) on her/his shoulder blades.

﹥ Gently pull the belt while the practitioner is curving her/his back and places the buttocks on the wall.

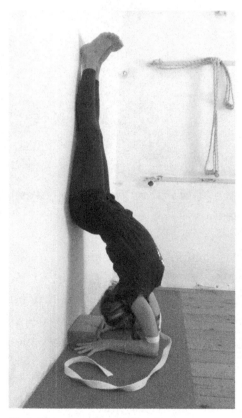

Pīncha Mayurāsana Viparīta Karaṇi

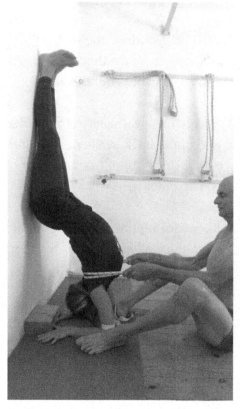

Pīncha Mayurāsana Viparīta Karaṇi with a helper

Viparīta Karaṇi

Variation 3
*Sirsāsana Viparīta Karaṇi:
Using the wall*

Effects
Creates movement in the shoulders region and opens the chest.

Props
wall, helper,
belt or rope

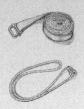

If you are supple, you can practice this Variation on your own, but a helper can improve the range of movement significantly; hence I describe it here as done with a helper.

Instructions for the practitioner:

→ Do *Sirsāsana* at about 40 cm (15 inches) away from the wall, and tilt back to have the heels supported by the wall.

Instructions for the helper:

> Once the practitioner is in the pose, sit in front of her/him. Place your feet against the elbows of the practitioner and a belt (or a rope) on his/her shoulder blades.

> Gently pull the belt while the practitioner is curving his/her back and places the buttocks on the wall.

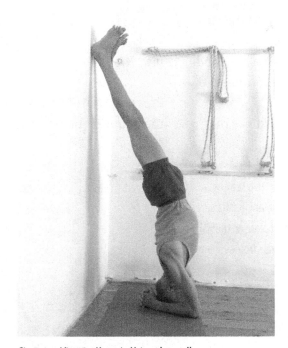

Sirsāsana Viparīta Karaṇi - Using the wall

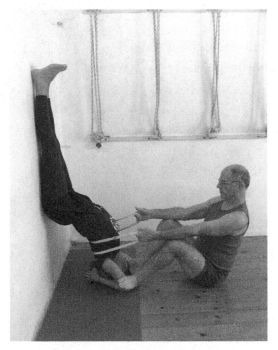

Sirsāsana Viparīta Karaṇi: with a helper

Variation 4
Sirsāsana Viparīta Karaṇi:
Using a chair

Effects
The chair support enables an extended stay in the pose, which has deep effects on the circulation and the breathing. The effects are somewhere between those of Sirsāsana and those of Dwi Pāda Viparīta Dandāsana.

Props
chair, blanket
(optional)

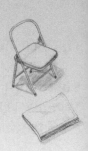

This Variation is less strenuous than the previous one, and hence you can stay in it longer. Still, it requires balance and flexibility in the shoulders and back.

⟶ Place a chair on a sticky mat

Notes:

1. If you are tall, raise the seat of the chair using several blankets. Be sure to place a sticky mat piece on the seat to prevent the blankets from slipping.

2. If the chair is too high for you, place a couple of folded blankets in front of the chair to raise the level of the floor.

❯ Sit on the chair and turn to place your legs on the backrest.

❯ Hold the chair and pull yourself toward the backrest until the pelvis is under the backrest.

❯ Now start to slide down from the chair; as you do so, arch the back such that the top of the head is descending toward the floor.

❯ Keep sliding until the top of the head rests on the mat (or on folded blanket placed on the mat).

❯ Release the backrest and move the hands down and form a cup-shape behind the head, as in *Sirsāsana.*

❯ Move the legs away from the backrest and stretch them vertically up.

❯ Press the forearms down, move the shoulder blades in and lift the shoulders.

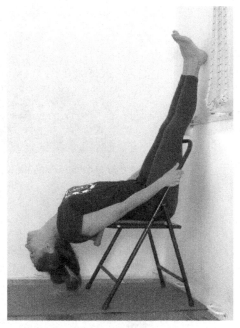

Entering *Sirsāsana Viparīta Karaṇi* with a chair

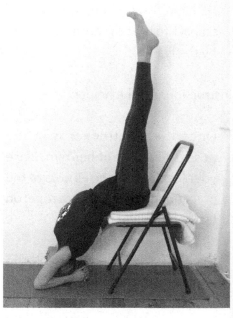

Sirsāsana Viparīta Karaṇi with a chair

Effects

Opens the chest and creates flexibility in the wrists. It is also a relaxing variation.

Sarvāṇgāsana Viparīta Karaṇi can be done with a chair (See Variation 16 on page 86) or a bench, but it can also be done by supporting the back with the palms. In this Variation one starts from *Sarvāṇgāsana* and arches the back to place the sacro-lumbar on the palms.

→ Prepare a platform for *Sarvāṇgāsana*, place the belt on your elbows and go up to *Sarvāṇgāsana* (see page 63).

❯ After staying a while in *Sarvāṇgāsana*, turn the palms such that the fingers point up (toward the buttocks).

❯ Then curve the upper back to descend the buttocks down.

❯ Support the back with the palms. Keep pressing the top shoulders down while lifting the upper back and shoulder blades.

❯ Stretch the legs vertically up. Relax and flatten the abdomen and breathe smoothly.

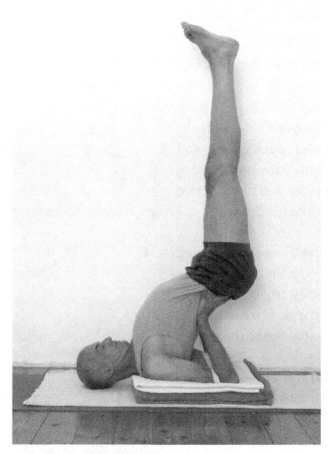

Independent *Sarvāṇgāsana Viparīta Karaṇi*

Viparīta Karaṇi

Variation 6
Restorative Viparīta Karaṇi: Using a block

This restorative Variation combines deep relaxation with opening of the chest. The harder support of the block moves the sacrum in and the increased height helps to release the pelvic region and to create space in the abdominal and chest cavities.

Props

block, wall, belt (optional)

In this Variation, a block supports the sacrum; the legs can rest on the wall, either held with a belt or stretched up independently.

⟶ Place the mat perpendicular to the wall and prepare the block next to it.

❭ Lie down on your side with the buttock bones touching the wall; then roll onto your back, taking your legs up the wall to supported Ūrdhva Prasārita Pādāsana ❶.

❭ Now push the feet against the wall to lift the pelvis up, and place the block about 25 cm (nearly a foot) away from the wall, standing with its wide side parallel to the wall.

❭ Curve to lift the upper back and roll onto the tops of the shoulders down.

❭ Then descend the sacrum to the block.

> **Note:** The height of the block should allow the buttocks to go down until the pelvis rests on it horizontally.

❭ Rest the legs against the wall ❷, hold the legs with a belt ❸, or stretch them vertically up ❹.

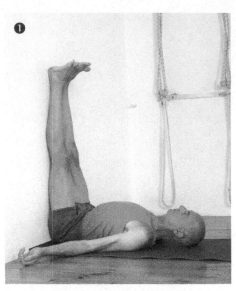

Lying in supported Ūrdhva Prasārita Pādāsana

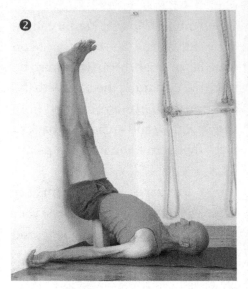

Viparīta Karaṇi: Using a block – legs on wall

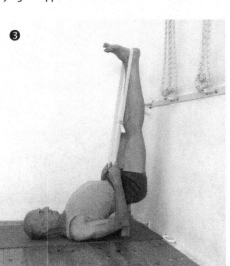

Viparīta Karaṇi: Using a block – holding the legs with a belt

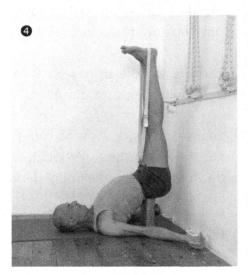

Viparīta Karaṇi: Using a block – stretching the legs

Tips

✔ Soften the inner groins and let them descend until the pubic bone is horizontal.

✔ You can do several leg variations as explained in the following Variation.

Viparīta Karaṇī

Variation 7
Deep Relaxation: Restorative Viparīta Karaṇī on a bolster

Effects

This restorative version of Viparīta Karaṇī is often called the "fountain of youth" because of its profound restorative effects. Few āsana-s have both the soothing and energizing effect of this Variation. It intensifies blood flow to the lymph nodes in the groins; this, combined with the deep relaxation, strengthens the immune system.

Props

block, 2-3 blankets, bolster, wall, belt

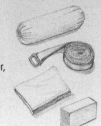

For most people, the standard bolster size is too narrow and too shallow for good opening for the chest, hence additional width and height should be added. A mat is used to prevent sliding away from the wall.

Preparation:

→ Place a mat perpendicular to the wall.

❯ Place a middle-height-block next to the wall.

> **Note:** The purpose of the block is to prevent the bolster from sliding toward the wall; a rolled blanket may also be used for this purpose.

❯ Fold a blanket into three and place it at about 30 cm (1 foot) away from the wall, such that when placing the bolster on it, it will slant slightly toward the wall; this will improve the support of the back during the pose ❶.

❯ Place the bolster next to the block ❷.

❯ If needed add another folded blanket on top of the bolster ❸.

❯ Place a belt near the bolster.

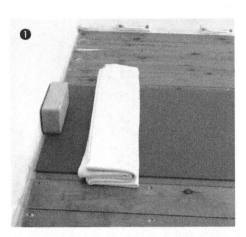
❶ Placing block and 3-folded blanket for *Viparīta Karaṇī*

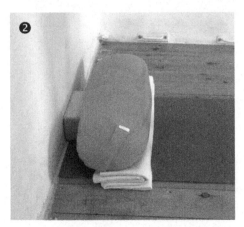
❷ Bolster on blanket

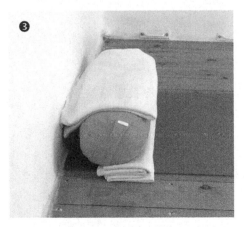
❸ Arrangement for supported *Viparīta Karaṇī*

Viparīta Karaṇi

Variation 7 (Cont'd)
Deep Relaxation:
Restorative Viparīta Karaṇi on a bolster

Entering the pose:

There are two ways to enter the pose: rolling sideways or rolling forward.

Rolling sideways:

⟶ Sit on the bolster with your side to the wall ❶.

❯ Roll to bring your buttock bones to the wall, taking your legs up the wall ❷.

❯ If the buttocks are not touching the wall, push the feet against the wall to lift the pelvis ❸. Then walk the shoulders toward the wall, lower the buttocks and feel the sitting bones touching the wall.

Rolling forward:

⟶ Stand in front of the bolster; bend forward and place the hands on the floor; now tuck the chin well in between the collar bones and roll forward ❹, supporting yourself with the palms until the shoulders rest safely on the bolster.

❯ Roll on the shoulders and lift the buttocks and the legs gently to the wall. Then slide down, descending the shoulders to the floor and the pelvis to the bolster ❺.

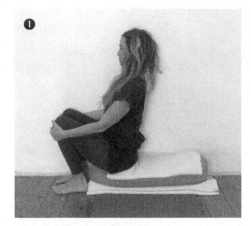
Sitting side to the wall

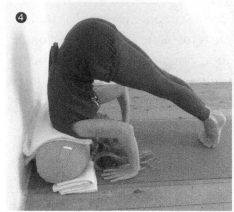
Rolling forward to *Viparīta Karaṇi*

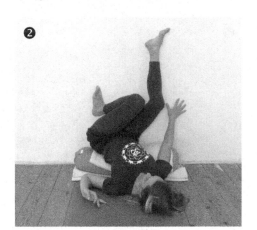
Rolling sideways to *Viparīta Karaṇi*

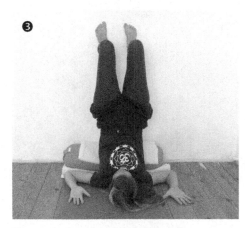
Moving the shoulders closer to the wall

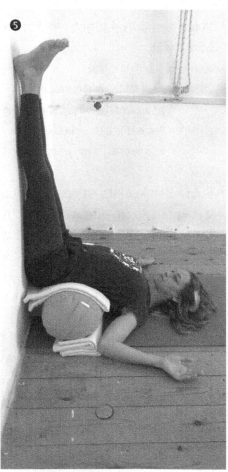
Restorative *Viparīta Karaṇi*

In the pose:

→ Curve the back to allow the sacral band to descend down in order to rest on the bolster.

❯ Keep the legs straight but relaxed, resting on the wall.

❯ Rest the arms on the floor and stay in the pose up to 25 minutes.

❯ Keep your eyes closed and observe your breath. Direct your attention to the breath and the internal sensations.

Option: Strap a belt around the top thighs. Make sure not to place the buckle on your skin.

Variations:

1. Legs crossed in *Swastikāsana* or *Padmāsana* ❶.

2. Legs bent to *Baddha Koṇāsana* ❷.

3. Legs spread as in *Upaviṣtha Koṇāsana* ❸. You can use the belt to support the feet ❹.

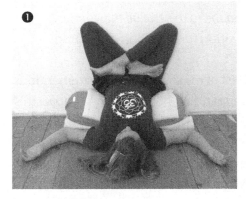
❶

Legs crossed in *Padmāsana*

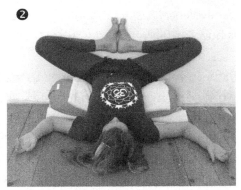
❷

Legs bent to *Baddha Koṇāsana*

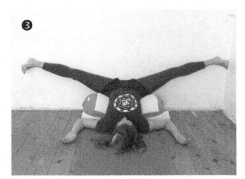
❸

Legs spread in *Upaviṣtha Koṇāsana*

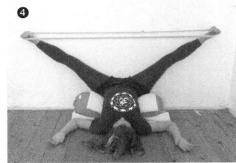
❹

Legs spread in *Upaviṣtha Koṇāsana* with belt

Coming out of the pose:

→ Slide down, away from the wall until the buttocks rest on the floor; cross the legs on the bolster or bend them in *Baddha Koṇāsana* (not shown).

❯ Stay a minute or two before rolling sideways and sitting.

Final words

"Yoga is for all. Nobody should be denied the opportunity to experience its benevolence. It is this thought that impelled me to think of all these props." – this is how Guruji Iyengar describes his motivation for developing the props.

In these volumes, I try to convey, to the best of my knowledge, the tremendous work done by Guruji and his deep understanding of the *āsana-s*. I hope this helps to spread this knowledge and make it more accessible for practitioners and teachers alike. The credit for all these innovations goes to Guruji, and if, when transmitting this knowledge, I unintentionally introduced errors, then he is not to blame, since it is because of my ignorance.

I hope you have enjoyed this journey as much as I have!

Appendix 3.1:
Vinyāsa – Practice sequences

. . . .

The effect of yoga practice is highly influenced by the order in which the *āsana-s* are performed in a particular session. This is called *Vinyāsa* or *Vinyāsakrama*. Correct sequencing is based on intimate knowledge of the energetic properties of each *āsana* and its anatomical, physiological, neurological, sensory and mental repercussions. The sequence is then selected according to the purpose and intention of the session; it takes into consideration one's practice experience and maturity, one's current physical and mental condition, the purpose of performing the sequence as well as the characteristics of the environment in which the practice takes place.

The effects of a sequence depend to a large extent on the position of the inverted poses in the sequence. This appendix presents four sequences with different purposes.

The **first sequence** is a 'standard' sequence, suitable for students at an intermediate level. *Sālamba Sirsāsana* is practiced after some energizing and opening *āsana-s* (standing poses, *Adho Mukha Śvānāsana* and *Adho Mukha Vṛksāsana*), and *Sālamba Sarvāngāsana* is practiced at the end, just before *Śavāsana*.

The **second sequence** is designed for more advanced practitioners, who already gained maturity in the practice of *Sirsāsana*. In this sequence *Sālamba Sirsāsana* is practiced as the first *āsana*, without any warm-ups. It is inspired by the sequences presented in *Light on Yoga* (from the 14th week onward). Starting with *Sirsāsana* quickly creates alertness and sharpness combined with coolness and passivity in the brain; it has a rather dramatic effect on the practice of the following *āsana-s* in the sequence.

The **third sequence** has a 'mirror structure,' in which *Sirsāsana* and *Sarvāngāsana* are framed within a progression of other *āsana-s*. In this case, these inverted *āsana-s* are done after some pacifying forward bends, which are then followed in the reverse order.

The **fourth sequence** is an example of how inverted *āsana-s* may be used as a preparation for *Prānāyāma* practice.

In case you want to perform these sequences when your time is short, you can shorten the duration of all the *āsana-s* in the sequence, without altering the proportions. For example, you can reduce the timings by staying in each *āsana* 50% or 75% of the given time.

For most *āsana-s*, a reference to the page number where the Variation appears, in this Volume or in the previous ones, is given. Explanatory comments are provided for the steps that are not included in the first three Volumes.

1. An Intermediate Level Sequence

**Characteristics
of this sequence are:**

> **Duration:** 75 min.

> **Level:** Intermediate

> **Type:** A 'standard' sequence

> **Types of *āsana-s* included:** Standing, Inversions

This is an intermediate level sequence which starts with some standing poses and shoulder openings, before moving to the inversions. *Supta Vīrāsana* is given as a relaxation between the active standing poses and the inversions which follow.

Props

**2 blocks, 5-6
blankets, belt,
wall**

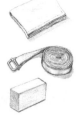

1. *Ūrdhva Hastāsana*

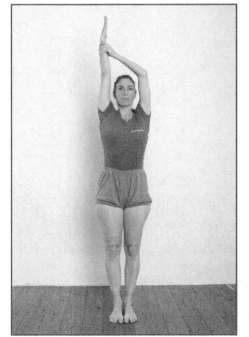

1 min.

See Vol. I, P. 20

2. *Ūrdhva Hastāsana - with blocks against wall*

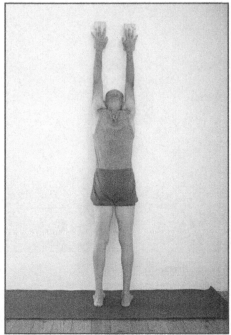

1 min.

See Vol. I, P. 22

3. *Adho Mukha Śvānāsana –* hands on blocks

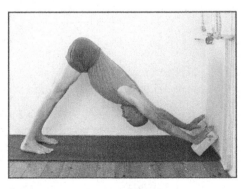

1 min.

See Vol. I, P. 32

4. *Adho Mukha Śvānāsana –*
feet on blocks

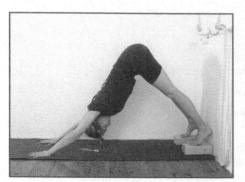

1 min.

See Vol. I, P. 39

5. *Utthita Trikonāsana –* top hand
holds weight

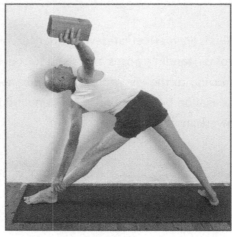

45 sec. on each side

See Vol. I, P. 90

6. *Virabhadrāsana II –* holding
a block

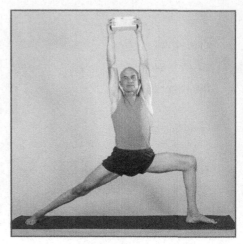

45 sec. on each side

See Vol. I, P. 102

7. *Virabhadrāsana I –* belt
around elbows

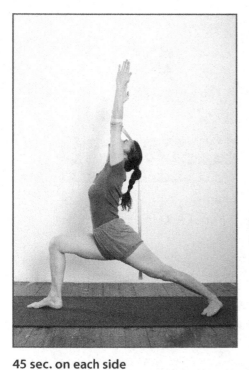

45 sec. on each side

See Vol. I, P. 112

8. *Virabhadrāsana I –* arms behind
the back

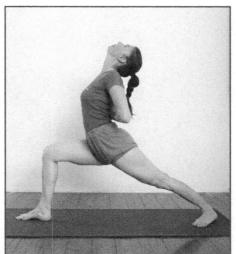

45 sec. on each side

See Vol. I, P. 115

9. *Uttānāsana –* arms behind
the back

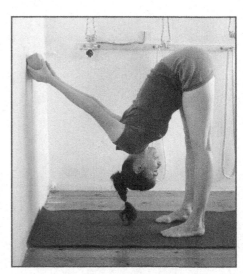

45 sec. × 2

See Vol. I, P. 64

10. *Supta Vīrāsana* - catching hooks

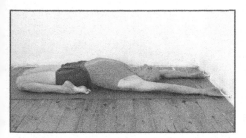

5 min.

Supta Vīrāsana can be done actively or restoratively.

Stretching to catch the hooks elongates the torso and reduces pressure from the lower back.

Alternatively, use a bolster to support the back and a blanket for the head and tighten a belt around the legs.

11. *Adho Mukha Vīrāsana* - belts on groins

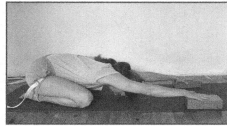

2 min.
See Vol. II, P. 75

12. *Adho Mukha Śvānāsana* – head support

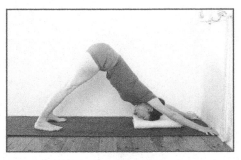

2 min.
See Vol. I, P. 51

13. *Adho Mukha Vṛkṣāsana* - hands on blocks

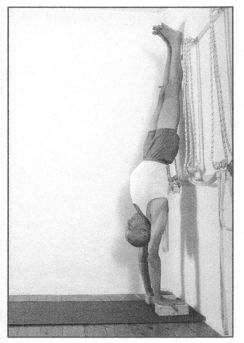

Hands forward, 45 sec.
See Vol. III, P. 127

14. *Adho Mukha Vṛkṣāsana* - hands on blocks

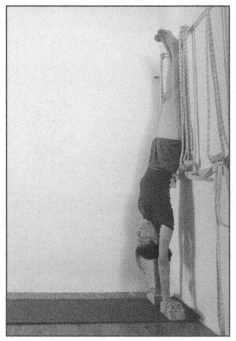

Hands sideways, 45 sec.
See Vol. III, P. 127

15. *Sālamba Sirsāsana I*

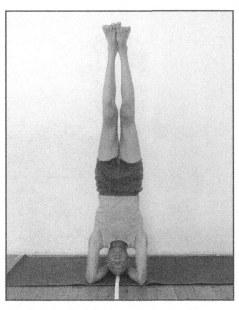

8 min.
See Vol. III, P. 18 or P. 19
Choose Variation 6 or 7, according to your needs

16. *Pārśva Sirsāsana*

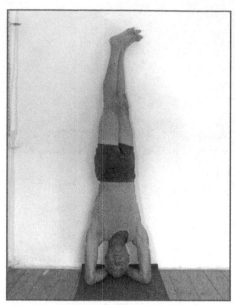

45 sec. each leg
See Vol. III, P. 45
Continue directly from *Sirsāsana*. You can use a wall to help maintain the alignment

17. *Pīncha Mayurāsana*

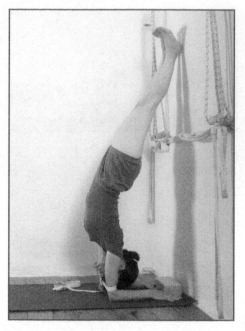

40 sec. × 2
See Vol. III, P. 112
palms against blocks

18. *Sālamba Sarvāngāsana I*

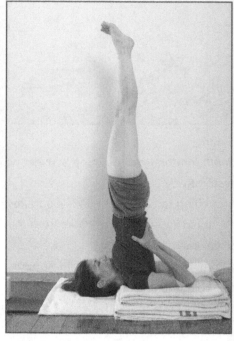

3 min.
See Vol. III, P. 64

19. *Halāsana* - belt on wrists

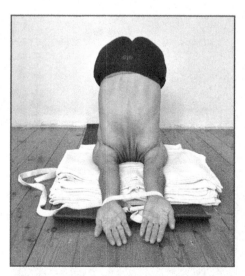

Shorten the loop of the belt and place it on the wrists
3 min.
See Vol. III, P. 90

20. *Karnapidāsana* - knees on blocks

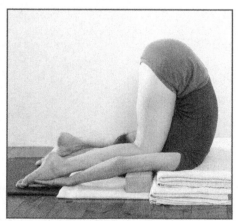

1 min.
See Vol. III, P. 94

21. *Sālamba Sarvāngāsana II*

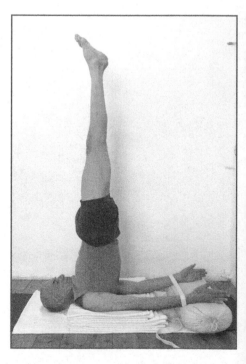

See Vol. III, P. 73

22. *Sālamba Sarvāngāsana I*

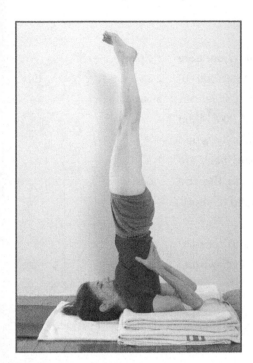

3 min.
See Vol. III, P. 64
....

23. *Setu Bandha Sarvāngāsana –* on block, feet against the wall

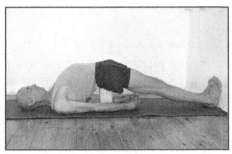

1 min.
See Vol. III, P. 147
....

24. *Adho Mukha Swastikāsana –* block support

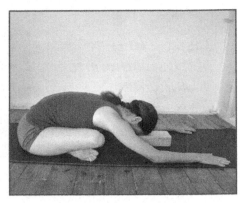

45 sec. each leg crossing

....

25. *Śavāsana* - with eye cover and block on abdomen

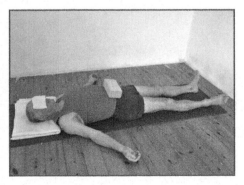

8-10 min.

....

2. Advanced Sequence: starting from *Sirsāsana*

Characteristics of this sequence are:

> **Duration:** 60 min.

> **Level:** Advanced

> **Type:** A '*Sirsāsana*-first' sequence, forward extensions using blocks

> **Types of *āsana-s* included:** Inversions, Forward extensions

This sequence starts from *Sirsāsana* – it is suitable for mature practitioners that can stay in *Sirsāsana* 10 minutes or more. If starting from *Sirsāsana* challenges you, then add some warming-up *āsana-s* (like *Adho Mukha Śvānāsana*) before *Sirsāsana*, especially when practicing in the morning. If your arms and neck are not strong enough and your body is not warm, then be careful not to strain your neck as this may lead to injury.

Sirsāsana is followed by standing and sitting forward bends, which are then followed by the *Sarvāngāsana* cycle.

Props
2 blocks, 5-6 blankets, belt

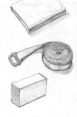

1. *Sālamba Sirsāsana I*

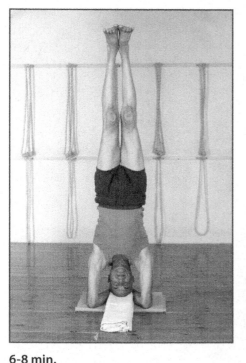

6-8 min.
See Vol. III, P. 23

2. *Pārśva Sirsāsana*

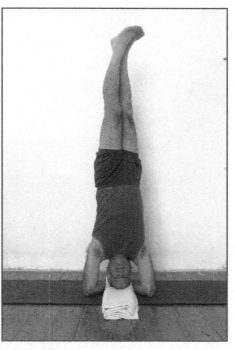

40-60 sec. each side
See Vol. III, P. 45

3. *Eka Pāda Sirsāsana*

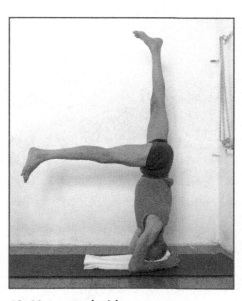

40-60 sec. each side
See Vol. III, P. 46

4. *Adho Mukha Vīrāsana* - belts on groins

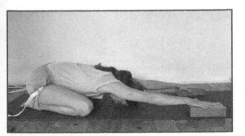

1 min.

See Vol. II, P. 75

5. *Uttānāsana* – back of legs against wall

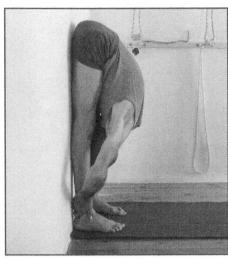

2 min.

See Vol. I, P. 57

6. *Prasārita Padottānāsana* - feet against wall and block

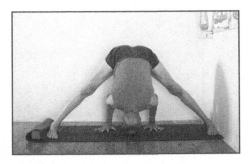

2 min.

See Vol. I, P. 139

7. *Adho Mukha Śvānāsana* – feet elevated

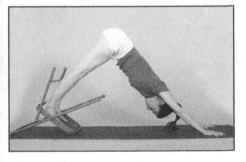

2 min.

See Vol. I, P. 39

8. *Uttānāsana* – head support

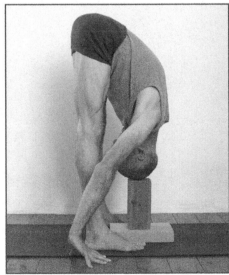

1 min.

See Vol. I, P. 66

9. *Paschimottānāsana* - holding blocks

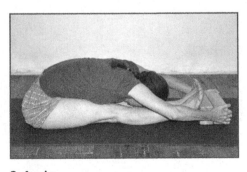

3-4 min.

See Vol. II, P. 99

10. *Jānu Sirsāsana* - holding block

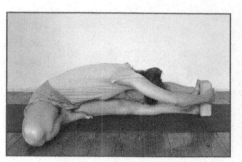

2 min. each side
See Vol. II, P. 127

11. *Ardha Padma Paschimottānāsana* - holding block

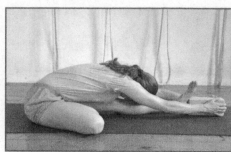

2 min. each side

12. *Paschimottānāsana* - elbows support

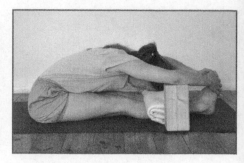

3-4 min.
See Vol. II, P. 112

13. *Bhardvajāsana I*

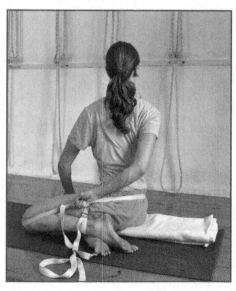

1 min. each side
See step 14 in Sequence 2 in Vol. 2, P. 147

14. *Sālamba Sarvāngāsana I*

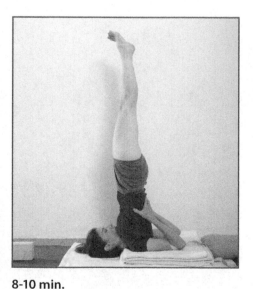

8-10 min.
See Vol. III, P. 64
Since the entire *Sarvāngāsana* cycle is done sequentially, adjust the platform next to the wall as explained in Variation 4 of *Setu Bandha Sarvāngāsana*

15. *Halāsana* - toes on block

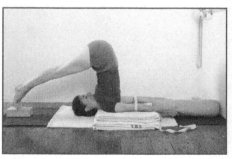

4-5 min.
See Vol. III, P. 63

16. *Karṇapīḍāsana* - knees on blocks

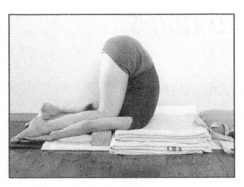

1 min.

See Vol. III, P. 94

17. *Supta Koṇāsana*

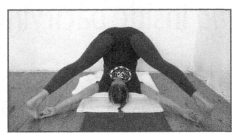

1 min.

18. *Setu Bandha Sarvāṅgāsana* - feet against wall

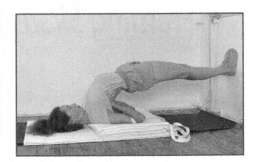

5 min.

See Vol. III, P. 102

19. *Śavāsana* - with eye cover and block on abdomen

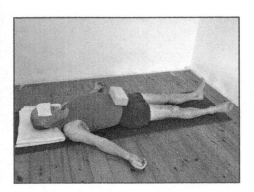

8-10 min.

3. Intermediate Sequence: Framing *Sirsāsana* inside pacifying *āsana-s*

Characteristics of this sequence are:

> **Duration:** 60 min.

> **Level:** Advanced

> **Type:** Cyclic ('mirror' structure)

> **Types of *āsana-s* included:** Inversions, Forward extensions

This sequence starts with standing and sitting forward bends followed by inverted *āsana-s*. The same forward bends are then repeated in the reverse order, which leads to a long *Tadāsana*. The pacifying forward bends quiet the brain and induce a pensive-meditative state. Repeating the same forward bends after the inversions strengthens this effect and allows for slow 'return' from the deep cooling effect. The final *Tadāsana*, which is done facing the wall, is a deep meditative practice.

The timings given are designed to induce deep unfolding and surrender. If you find it too demanding, you can still follow this sequence by decreasing the timings.

To avoid disturbing the flow, it is recommended to prepare the platform for *Sarvāngāsana* in advance.

Props

2 blocks, 5-6 blankets, belt

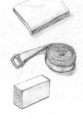

---

1. *Uttānāsana* - head support

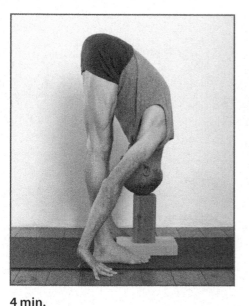

4 min.
See Vol. I, P. 66

2. *Adho Mukha Śvānāsana* - head support

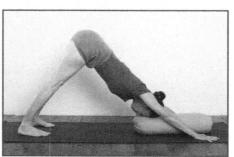

4 min.
See Vol. I, P. 52

3. *Prasārita Padottānāsana* - feet against wall and block

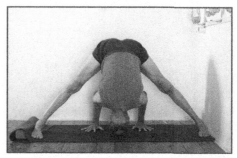

4 min.
See Vol. I, P. 139

If the head does not rest on the floor, support it with a folded blanket or block

4. *Jānu Sirsāsana* - holding block

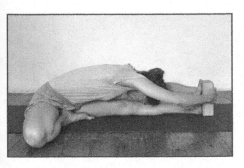

2 min. each side
See Vol. II, P. 127

5. *Paschimottānāsana* - holding block

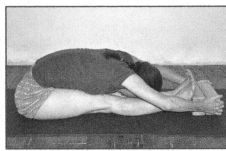

4 min.
See Vol. II, P. 99

6. *Adho Mukha Vīrāsana* - belts on groins

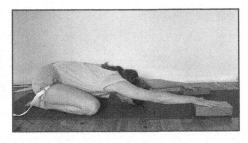

1 min.
See Vol. II, P. 75

7. *Sālamba Sirsāsana I*

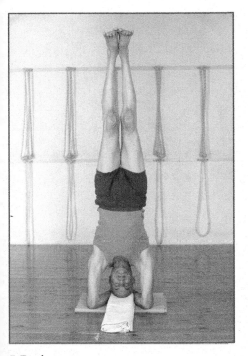

5-7 min.
See Vol. III, P. 23

8. *Sālamba Sarvāngāsana I*

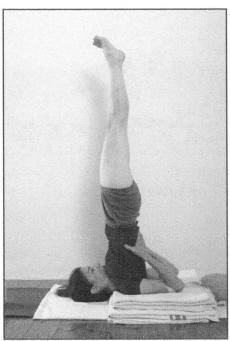

7-8 min.
See Vol. III, P. 64

9. *Halāsana* - toes on block

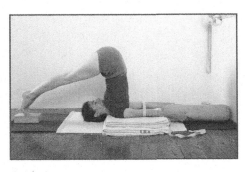

4 min.
See Vol. III, P. 63

10. *Karnapidāsana* - knees on blocks

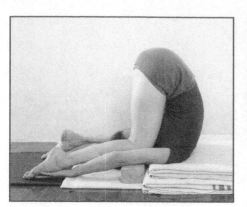

1 min.
See Vol. III, P. 94

11. *Supta Koṇāsana*

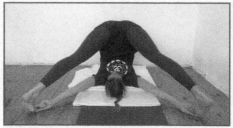

1 min.
You can use 2 chairs as in Vol. III, P. 89

12. *Setu Bandha Sarvāngāsana* - with wide support

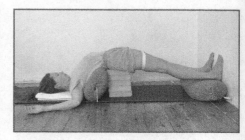

5 min.
See Vol. III, P. 105

13. *Adho Mukha Vīrāsana* - belts on groins

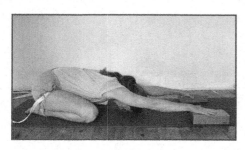

1 min.
See Vol. II, P. 78

14. *Paschimottānāsana* - holding block

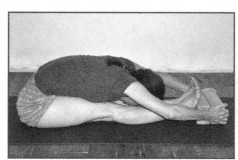

4 min.
See Vol. II, P. 99

15. *Jānu Sirsāsana* - holding block

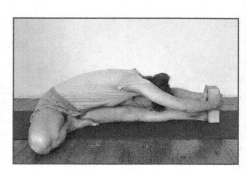

2 min. each side
See Vol. II, P. 127

16. *Prasārita Pādōttānāsana -* feet against wall and block

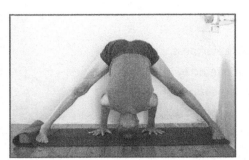

2 min.

See Vol. I, P. 139

If the head does not rest on the floor, support it with a folded blanket or block

17. *Adho Mukha Śvānāsana* - head support

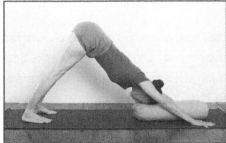

4 min.

See Vol. I, P. 52

18. *Uttānāsana* - head support

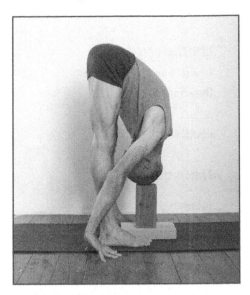

4 min.

See Vol. I, P. 66

19. *Tadāsana* - facing a wall

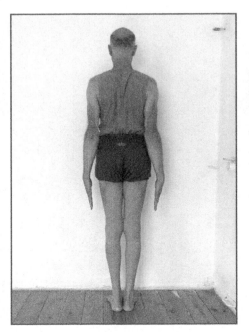

5 min.

Stand facing the wall at about 20 cm (8 inches) away from it

20. *Śavāsana* - lower legs on chair

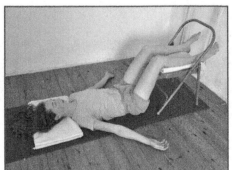

7-10 min.

4. Pacifying Sequence: Inversions for *Prāṇāyāma*

Characteristics of this sequence are:

> **Duration:** 90 min.

> **Level:** Advanced

> **Type:** Restorative

> **Types of *āsana-s* included:** Inversions, Forward extensions

The inverted *āsana-s* open the chest and create alertness and passivity and hence prepare the body and mind for *Prāṇāyāma*. In this sequence props are used to support and pacify. After about 50 minutes of restorative *āsana-s*, one is ready for supported *Śavāsana* which is the starting point for *Prāṇāyāma*. If sitting *Prāṇāyāma* is too challenging, be satisfied with reclining *Prāṇāyāma*. As you advance in the practice of *āsana-s* you will find that sitting becomes approachable.

Props

2 blocks, 5-6 blankets, 1-2 belts, wall hook or door handle

1. *Adho Mukha Śvānāsana* - with rope and head support

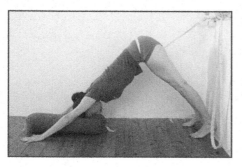

3 min.
See Vol. I, P. 53-4

2. *Uttānāsana* – with rope

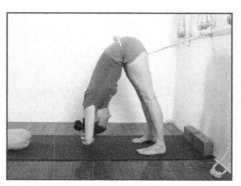

2 min.
See Vol. I, P. 54

3. *Uttānāsana* – head support

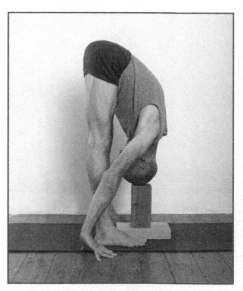

3 min.
See Vol. I, P. 66

4. *Prasārita Padottānāsana* - feet against wall and block

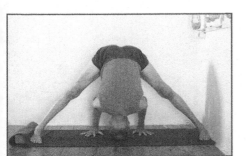

2 min.

See Vol. I, P. 139

If the head does not rest on the floor, support it with a folded blanket or block

5. *Sirsāsana* - from rope

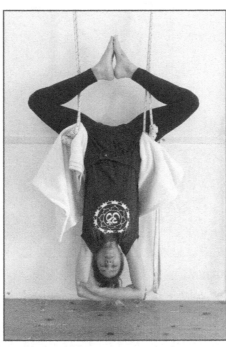

8 min.

See Vol. III, P. 59

6. *Viparīta Dandāsana* - on cross bolsters or bench

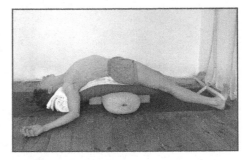

5 min.

See Vol. III, P. 6

7. *Sarvāngāsana* - from chair

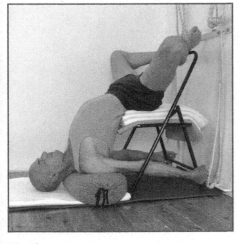

10 min.

See Vol. III, P. 87

8. *Setu bandha Sarvāngāsana* - on bolster

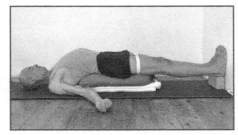

6 min.

See Vol. III, P. 106

9. *Supta Baddha Konāsana* - with bolster and crossed belt on feet

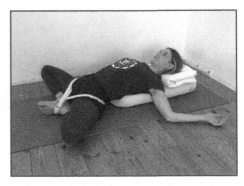

5 min.

10. *Śavāsana Prāṇāyāma* - on bolster or blocks

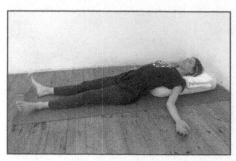

10 min.

Start with *Ujjai I*, and gradually proceed to *Ujjai II* and *Viloma I* (see *Light on Prāṇāyāma*)

....

11. Sitting *Prāṇāyāma* - with knees supportt

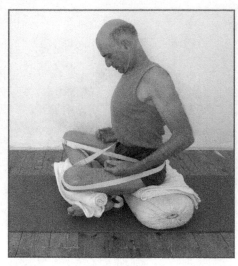

10 min.
See Vol. II, P. 35

....

12. *Śavāsana* - with eye cover and block on abdomen

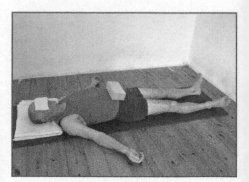

8 min.

....

Index:

> If applicable, the Variation number (e.g. V. 5) is given after the keyword.

> Note that the Variation number is of the corresponding *āsana*.

> Sub-entries are ordered according to the word whose initial is capitalized.

· ·

Made in the USA
Monee, IL
30 March 2022

93821714R00103